AIDS
AND INTRAVENOUS
DRUG USE

AIDS AND INTRAVENOUS DRUG USE

Community Intervention and Prevention

Edited by

C. G. Leukefeld
R. J. Battjes
Z. Amsel
Division of Clinical Research
National Institute on Drug Abuse

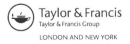

Taylor & Francis
Taylor & Francis Group
LONDON AND NEW YORK

This permanent edition contains the complete text of the National Institute on Drug Abuse's report, *AIDS and Intravenous Drug Use: Future Directions for Community-Based Prevention Research.* This work was the product of a review meeting sponsored by the division of Clinical Research, National Institute of Drug Abuse.

First published by Hemisphere Publishing Corporation

This edition published 2012 by Taylor & Francis

27 Church Road, Hove, East Sussex BN3 2FA

711 Third Avenue, New York, NY 10017

Taylor & Francis is an imprint of the Taylor & Francis Group, an informa business

AIDS AND INTRAVENOUS DRUG USE: Community Intervention and Prevention

Cover design by Sharon M. DePass.
A CIP catalog record for this book is available from the British Library.

Library of Congress Cataloging-in-Publication Data

AIDS and intravenous drug use : community intervention and prevention
  / edited by C. G. Leukefeld, R. J. Battjes, Z. Amsel.
      p.   cm.
    Originally published in 1990 by U.S. Dept. of Health and Human
  Services, Public Institute on Drug Abuse, and Mental Health
  Administration, National Institute on Drug Abuse, Rockville, Md.
    Includes bibliographical references and index.

    1. AIDS (Disease)—Prevention.   2. Narcotic addicts—Diseases.
  I. Leukefeld, Carl G.   II. Battjes, Robert.   III. Amsel, Z.
  RA644.A25A3459   1990
  616.97'9205—dc20   90-37065
                                                                CIP

  ISBN 1-56032-141-5

Contents

Introducing the Concept "Community Prevention"

Zili Amsel, Sc.D.

The impact of the acquired immunodeficiency syndrome (AIDS) on intravenous (IV) drug abusers is only beginning to be assessed. According to the surveillance system of the Centers for Disease Control (CDC), over 25 percent of all reported adult and adolescent cases of AIDS in the United States are attributed to IV drug abuse, and the percentage is growing (Centers for Disease Control 1988). However, the effect of AIDS on IV drug abusers has been even greater than indicated by AIDS case data. Many IV drug abusers have died of AIDS-related conditions. AIDS among heterosexual IV drug abusers has been reported in all 50 States, the District of Columbia, and Puerto Rico, and is heavily concentrated along the East Coast. For women with AIDS, IV drug abuse is the primary risk factor, accounting for 52 percent of adult and adolescent female cases. Finally, 11 percent of gay AIDS cases also have IV drug abuse as a risk factor.

Ethnic groups, overrepresented among IV drug abusers, are also overrepresented among heterosexual IV drug abusers with AIDS. Whereas blacks account for 12 percent of the U.S. population, blacks make up 51 percent of heterosexual IV drug abusers with AIDS. Similarly, while 6 percent of the general population are Hispanic, over 30 percent of the heterosexual IV drug abusers with AIDS are Hispanic.

According to reports from the National Institute on Drug Abuse (NIDA), there are an estimated 1.1 to 1.3 million IV drug abusers in the United States (Centers for Disease Control 1987). Various studies (Lange et al. 1988; Des Jarlais et al. 1988a) report that between 70 percent and nearly 100 percent of IV drug abusers share the use of injection equipment, with resulting high risk for contracting and transmitting AIDS.

The effects of AIDS are not limited to IV drug abusers, but extend also to their sexual partners and children. About 70 percent of those born in the United States and reported to the CDC as having AIDS attribute their infection to heterosexual contact with an IV drug abuser. About 75 percent of perinatal transmission (from mother to child during pregnancy or childbirth) has been attributed to children of IV-drug-using women or to women who were the sexual partners of IV drug abusers (Chamberland et al. 1987; Oxtoby, personal communication, 1987).

Preventing the AIDS epidemic associated with IV drug abuse requires a broad program that includes multiple strategies. This effort must include interventions designed to alter high-risk behaviors among IV drug abusers and their sexual partners and to educate the public about the infection so that when a vaccine or therapeutic inter-vention becomes available, mechanisms are in place to reach those with the greatest need.

Risk-reduction programming needs to extend beyond medical and drug abuse treatment facilities to also reach IV drug abusers who are not in treatment and their sexual partners. These efforts need to include all sexual partners of IV drug abusers, not only spouses. It seems that AIDS prevention programs should separate components that disseminate information from those that are designed to change behaviors. Each of these approaches addresses different objectives, but they are interdependent, one approach reinforcing the other.

For the first approach, factual information about infection with the human immunodeficiency virus (HIV) and AIDS is provided through one or more channels, such as electronic media, written materials, or information sessions. For some people, information dissemination is sufficient to alter attitudes and behaviors. Usually, these are individuals who hold values and beliefs that are compatible with the messages being transmitted. The social networks of these individuals also support these messages and the associated behavior change. In most cases, those most readily affected by media messages are highly educated and mainstream members of the population. For any large-scale health promotion effort, however, messages channeled through media provide the structural support for more intensive behavior-change programs. Continued messages reinforce the norms of the community for the desired behaviors.

For harder-to-reach populations, particularly those not in the mainstream of society, such as addicted, needle-using persons, additional strategies are necessary. These strategies need to be tailored to address the special parameters of the target population. These parameters include perceptions of AIDS, its transmission, and its relative importance in the lives of the population, as well as existing levels of involvement in high-risk behaviors. Barriers and enhancers to the initiation and maintenance of desired behaviors also should be identified and addressed.

However, most educational programs directed towards AIDS prevention among IV drug abusers are concerned with information dissemination. Community outreach workers or professional workers intervene in one-on-one relationships and through informal contact and counseling to address the individual drug user's attitudes and behaviors. Many of these program activities are not standardized or well documented, making their assessment difficult to conduct.

Early studies conducted in New York and San Francisco have indicated that high levels of knowledge about AIDS exist among IV drug abusers (Des Jarlais et al. 1988b). Yet, knowledge alone does not appear to be sufficient incentive for individual behavior change. In interviews with 59 methadone patients in Manhattan regarding their knowledge of AIDS and their use of protective behaviors, Friedman and associates found that more than 90 percent were knowledgeable about AIDS (Friedman et al. 1986). However, only 54 percent reported any change in their drug injection practices.

In conjunction with a seroprevalence study conducted in 1984 and 1985 in New Jersey, an assessment was made of knowledge of AIDS and self-reported protective behaviors among IV drug abusers in treatment. Facts about AIDS, how HIV is transmitted, and its symptoms were well known to these IV drug abusers. However, knowledge was not related to behavior change, and only about one-third of those interviewed knew how to sterilize injection equipment. Furthermore, about a third incorrectly believed that those infected with HIV necessarily show signs and symptoms of infection. Finally, slightly more than half were aware that HIV could be transmitted sexually or perinatally (Ginzburg et al. 1986).

Educational programs have had some success in changing drug injection behavior and in enrolling abusers in drug treatment programs. For example, in San Francisco, local health outreach workers are distributing small bottles of bleach and instructions for cleaning injection equipment. During the period prior to the program, 3 percent of IV drug abusers interviewed as part of an evaluation study reported that they used bleach for this purpose. One year later, 67 percent reported that they did so (Watters et al. 1987). In New Jersey, outreach workers developed a voucher system for treatment programs for those IV drug abusers who could not pay for such services. The vouchers served three purposes: (1) to measure contacts on the street, (2) to describe the characteristics of those reached, and (3) to facilitate entry into treatment. It was found that 80 percent of the first 1,000 vouchers were redeemed at detoxification programs. Of those redeeming vouchers, 40 percent had not previously been enrolled in treatment. After detoxification, over 200 individuals went on to longer treatment programs (Jackson et al., in press).

These reports indicate that providing information about AIDS risk factors alone has not been effective in altering high-risk behaviors. Thus, intervention programs must go beyond just providing facts and include behavior-change strategies that not only encourage the initiation of risk reduction, but also the maintenance of these behaviors. However, AIDS prevention strategies for IV drug abusers will not be directly comparable to those used for other AIDS risk groups, such as gay men and hemophilia and transfusion patients. Components from these programs, as well as from other types of programs such as those directed to smoking cessation, seat belt use, family planning, and cardiovascular disease and cancer prevention, can be incorporated into a comprehensive intervention model.

IV drug use is not a problem of one group but includes people from all social classes, educational levels, ethnic groups, religions, and geographic areas. The possession of drugs for nonmedical purposes is illegal throughout the United States, and possession of injection equipment is also illegal in most States. IV drug abuse has been found to be associated with other illegal or deviant behaviors (Des Jarlais et al. 1986; Des Jarlais et al. 1988a; Agar 1973). It should be recognized that for some persons and groups, drug abuse is inter- twined with their economic and social lives. Furthermore, sexual behavior, independent of IV drug use, is defined by group norms and individual sexual identity. Therefore, many personal, social, and cultural barriers must be addressed in order to alter high-risk drug use and sexual behaviors.

Because of the special needs of IV drug abusers and their sexual partners, an AIDS intervention program designed for this population should address multiple objectives and requires multilevel, highly integrated interventions. It is suggested here that the intervention should be community based to be effective in reaching the greatest numbers of the target population, particularly any hidden population such as the IV drug abuser not in drug abuse treatment programs. Such interventions should be designed to: (a) prepare various members of the community for forthcoming AIDS preventive efforts, (b) overcome barriers to high-risk-behavior change, and (c) bring about high-risk-behavior change among those in the community. Community support for AIDS-prevention programming suggests strategies that use multiple community channels, such as broadcast and print media. The media could be used to increase knowledge levels about HIV transmission and perceptions of susceptibility among residents. Messages for the general population should be clear, simple, to the point, and repeated. Human-interest stories about HIV infection could be presented to demonstrate that the problem is not limited to stereotypical drug abusers, but affects various people, their sexual partners, and their children, with whom drug abusers can identify. Eliminating the barrier between "them" and "us" will increase perceptions of individual susceptibility and familiarity, and redefine the AIDS problem as "our problem." A media program could be developed not just to reach drug abusers but also those around them to create an environment that encourages and reinforces behavior change. To assure support from the community, participation by leaders with broad constituencies is recommended, including religious groups, labor organizations, and political figures, as well as the involvement of local community leaders on active task forces and work groups.

Results of the Stanford and North Karelia cardiovascular disease prevention programs (Fortmann et al. 1986; Puska et al. 1983) suggest that behavior-change interventions should not only build on media support but also should focus on small group and individual interventions based on a theoretical framework. Printed or audiovisual materials along with personal discussions provide instructions for skills needed for behavior change as well as answer questions that arise in response to the educational messages. Furthermore, group sessions provide the social and psychological support needed for initiating and reinforcing such changes. It is suggested that groups identified with broad health, social, and community issues be used to help increase effectiveness. Finally, to reach those who are more self-directed or who have no social supports, interventions should include "one-on-one" strategies such as hotlines and counseling services.

A key resource that can fit within the context of a community-based prevention and intervention program is drug treatment, with aftercare components to reinforce the decision to give up drug use. Facilities for HIV testing and counseling, with followup and medical care, also must be available.

To identify and describe innovative ways for preventing and reducing the spread of HIV among drug abusers, their sexual partners, and their children, NIDA convened a technical review meeting in February 1988. The aim of the meeting was to propose recommendations for future directions for community-based prevention research within the context presented here. "Community," for the technical review, was defined as "any set of formal or informal group relationships that has some established criteria for membership." The chapters in this volume examine communities from two perspectives: (1) having one or more demographic characteristics, and (2) formal institutional membership. Each author was asked to describe current knowledge about HIV infection in a selected community; community factors or characteristics that support or hinder performance of protective and preventive behaviors (e.g., cultural, social, economic, psychological, or functional); any available documented community experiences specific to the target group with other related preventive behaviors; anecdotal experiences specific to the target group with behaviors associated with HIV transmission as well as other related preventive behaviors; suggestions for intervention models for the target groups; and suggestions for associated research initiatives.

Communities represented here include IV drug abusers who are black, Puerto Rican, and members of other Hispanic groups; white males; gays; users of nonopiate drugs; and prostitutes. Also incorporated are institutional settings, including schools, drug abuse treatment facilities, the criminal justice system, shelters for the homeless, the social service system, and the health care system.

Based on the papers presented, participants at the technical review meeting considered future directions in community AIDS prevention in two concurrent discussion groups focused on intervention models and research methodology. The recommendations of these groups are presented as the final chapter in this book.

REFERENCES

Agar, M.H. *Ripping and Running: A Formal Ethnography of Urban Heroin Addicts.* New York: Seminar Press, 1973. 79 pp.

Centers for Disease Control. Acquired immunodeficiency syndrome (AIDS). *Weekly Surveillance Report,* June 20, 1988.

Centers for Disease Control. *A Review of Current Knowledge and Plans for Expansion of HIV Surveillance Activities: A Report to the Domestic Policy Council.* November 30, 1987. 48 pp.

Chamberland, M.; White, C.; Lifson, A.; and Dondero, T.J. AIDS in heterosexual contacts: A small but interesting group of cases. Presented at the Third International Conference on AIDS, Washington, DC, June 1-5, 1987.

Des Jarlais, D.C.; Friedman, S.R.; Sothern, J.L.; and Stoneburner, R. The sharing of drug injection equipment and the AIDS epidemic in New York City: The first decade. In: Battjes, R.J., and Pickens, R.W., eds. *Needle Sharing Among Intravenous Drug Abusers: National and International Perspectives.* National Institute on Drug Abuse Research Monograph 80. DHHS Pub. No. (ADM)88-1567. Washington, DC: Supt. of Docs., U.S. Govt. Print. Off., 1988a. pp. 160-174.

Des Jarlais, D.C.; Friedman, S.R.; and Stoneburner, R.L. HIV infection and intravenous drug use: Critical issues in transmission dynamics, infection outcomes, and prevention. *Rev Infect Dis* 10:151-158, 1988b.

Des Jarlais, D.C.; Friedman, S.R.; and Strug, D. AIDS among intravenous drug users: A socio-cultural perspective. In: Feldman, D.A., and Johnson, T.A., eds. *Social Dimensions of AIDS: Methods and Theory.* New York: Praeger Publishing Company, 1986. pp. 11-126.

Fortmann, S.P.; Haskell, W.L.; Williams, P.T.; Varady, A.N.; Hulley, A.B.; and Farquhar, J.W. Community surveillance of cardiovascular disease in the Stanford Five-City Project: Methods and initial experience. *Am J Epidemiol* 123(4):656-669, April 1986.

Friedman, S.R.; Des Jarlais, D.C.; and Sothern, J.L. AIDS health education for intravenous drug users. *Health Educ Q* 13:383-393, 1986.

Ginzburg, H.M.; French, J.; Jackson, J.; Hartsock, P.I.; MacDonald, M.G.; and Weiss, S.H. Health education and knowledge assessment of HTLV-III diseases among intravenous drug users. *Health Educ Q* 13:373-382, 1986.

Jackson, J.; Rotkiewicz, L.G.; Quinones, M.A.; and Passannante, M.R. A coupon program: Drug treatment and AIDS education. *Int J Addict* 24, in press.

Lahge, W.R., et al. Geographic distribution of human immuno-deficiency virus markers in parenteral drug abusers. *Am J Public Health* 78(4):443-446, April 1988.

Oxtoby, M.J. Centers for Disease Control, personal communication, 1987.

Puska, P.; Salonen, J.A.; Nissinen, A.; Tuomilehto, J.; Vartiainen, E.; Korhonen, H.; Tanskanen, A.; Rönnqvist, P.; Koskela, K.; and Huttunen, J. Change in risk factors for coronary heart disease during 10 years of a community intervention programme. (North Karelia Project) *Br Med J* 287:1840-1844, 1983.

Watters, J.K. Preventing human immunodeficiency virus contagion among intravenous drug users: The impact of the street-based education on risk behavior. Presented at the Third International Conference on AIDS, Washington, DC, 1987.

AUTHOR

Zili Amsel, Sc.D.
Division of Clinical Research
National Institute on Drug Abuse
Parklawn Building, Room 10A16
5600 Fishers Lane
Rockville, MD   20857

Communication and Health Education Research: Potential Sources for Education for Prevention of Drug Use

Nathan Maccoby

INTRODUCTION

In this paper, research conducted during the last 20 years is briefly described that has been applied to reduction of disease risk in communities. Most of the work reported is based on the Stanford Center for Research in Disease Prevention's work in communities. Included are experiences from the Three Community Study (TCS), the still ongoing Five City Project (FCP), and the work done in schools. The hope is that some of this experience may suggest methods and ideas that might be successful in preventing or reducing behavior that may contribute to high risk of acquired immunodeficiency syndrome (AIDS) infection.

BACKGROUND

Chronic disease, especially cardiovascular disease (CVD) and, to a lesser extent, cancer, became the largest contributors to death and disability in this and other highly developed countries by the middle of this century. Risk factors for heart disease had been identified through the long-term Framingham study and other epidemiological investigations (Dawber 1980). The three major risk factors are smoking, high blood pressure, and blood cholesterol. As blood pressure and blood cholesterol could be controlled through diet, exercise, and drugs, it was seen that behavior changes needed to take place to reduce the risk of heart disease.

To address the prevention of CVD, John W. Farquhar and Stanford Medical School co-researchers Peter D. Wood, Byron W. Brown, Jr., William Haskell, and Michael Stern joined in a decision in early 1970 to develop a research plan to explore efficient means of risk

1

reduction in the population at large and to participate in clinical trials. In Farquhar's view, such a plan would require a broad inter-disciplinary team of biomedical and social scientists to address the wide range of questions raised by the research problem. This led him to reach beyond medical science and to consult with Nathan Maccoby, the Department of Communication, and other behavioral scientists. This group began to assess how best to design a public education program in CVD risk reduction.

Since the primary risk factors of smoking, diet, and high blood pres-sure were distributed across large segments of the total adult popula-tion, techniques that would reach large numbers of people were called for. At this point, the idea of intervening in total communities through mass media was introduced. After reviewing the projected limitations in resources and manpower, the decision was reached to limit the target population to all adults aged 35 to 59.

As a result of interaction between the communication researchers, psychologists, communication specialists, and others, Farquhar and the biomedical scientists made a basic change in the research plan. They turned from a medical model, concerned with high-risk populations and key health-professional opinion leaders, to a more complex but potentially more effective community model, relying principally on communication as the basic intervention tool.

The role of mass media in achieving behavior change is complex. Steve Chaffee, in a 1982 review of the evidence arguing that inter-personal sources of information are by nature more persuasive than media, points out that the evidence varies greatly (Chaffee 1982). Furthermore, mass media interact in complex ways with other sources of communication. Media information may lead one to seek inter-personal confirmation; the reverse is also true. For example, when people heard of the J.F. Kennedy assassination from others, they checked the truth of the rumor by consulting radio, TV, and newspapers.

Diffusion of information and practices takes place partly through mass media ("everybody is doing it"), and partly through institutions and organized groups. Communities can take on major tasks like pre-vention, using a myriad of facilities to organize activities. Schools, worksites, churches, clubs, and families can all serve as agents of a communitywide effort to achieve changes in behavior that puts people at risk or to prevent such behavior from being learned and performed.

The environment can be altered in ways that are likely to reduce the incidence of risky activities. Cigarette machines kept away from minors or abolished; smoking banned in worksites and public places; cigarette advertising banned or heavily restricted; more healthful foods supplanting disease-promoting ones in schools, restaurants, fast-food places, and food-dispensing machines all help to reduce the incidence of smoking and high-cholesterol diets. In addition, exercise opportunities can be made readily available to the public.

Since the media campaign was to be directed at entire communities, random assignment of individuals to the treatment or control condition was not feasible. An equally rigorous experimental method, treating a large number of entire, geographically defined populations as single units and randomly assigning some of these communities to treatment and some to control conditions, was not administratively possible (Farquhar 1978). We concluded that the most realistic compromise between feasibility and rigor was a quasi-experimental research approach using a small number of communities as experimental units.

After considering the powerful cultural forces that reinforce and maintain the health habits we wished to change, and in view of past failure of health education campaigns, we designed a heretofore untested combination of extensive mass media with a considerable amount of face-to-face instruction. We chose the latter method not so much because it was potentially widely applicable, but because it was judged most likely to succeed (Maccoby and Alexander 1979). It was then possible to compare mass media, a more generally applicable though less promising treatment with a sound approach. Therefore, another community was selected in which treatments were administered via mass media alone. Three strategies not usually incorporated in health campaigns were used in our approach:

(1)   the mass media materials were devised to teach specific behavioral skills, as well as to perform the more usual tasks of offering information and affecting attitudes and motivation;

(2)   both the mass media and, in particular, the face-to-face instruction were designed to embody many previously validated methods of achieving changes in behavior and self-control training principles; and

3

(3)   the campaign was designed on the basis of careful analysis of the specific needs and the media consumption patterns of the intended audiences. Our goal was to devise and evaluate methods for effecting changes in smoking, exercise, and diet that would be both cost effective and applicable to large population groups.

THE STANFORD THREE COMMUNITY STUDY (TCS)

Three roughly comparable communities in northern California were selected for the study. Tracy was chosen as a reference town because it was relatively distant and isolated from media in the other two communities. Gilroy and Watsonville, the other two communities, share some media channels (television and radio), but each town has its own newspaper. Watsonville and Gilroy received different strategies of health education over a period of 2 years. Both received health education through the mass media, but in Watsonville face-to-face was added using a randomized design with a sample of persons at high levels of risk for cardiovascular disease. Two-thirds of this group received the face-to-face instruction, while the remaining people in this group were exposed only to media health education.

The intensive instruction program was composed of education and persuasion in the context of social learning and self-control training procedures designed to achieve the same changes in cholesterol and fat consumption, body weight, cigarette smoking (Meyer et al. 1977), and physical exercises that were advocated in the media campaign. The instruction was conducted by a team of graduate students in communication, medical students, and health educators trained in behavior modification techniques. The protocols were pretested in a controlled setting before being applied in the field. The basic sequential strategy was to present information about the behavior that influences risk of coronary heart disease, stimulate personal analysis of existing behavior, and demonstrate desired skills (e.g., food selection and preparation), using such channels as TV spots and bus cards.

The mass media component consisted of a broad range of materials, including about 50 different television spots, 3 hours of television programming, over 100 different radio spots, several hours of radio programming, weekly newspaper columns, newspaper advertisements and stories, billboards, printed material sent via direct mail to participants, posters, and other assorted materials. Because of the sizable Spanish-speaking population in the communities, the campaign was

4

presented in both Spanish and English. The Spanish media programs were designed to be culturally relevant.

The dominant characteristic of the mass media campaign was organizational. The campaign was an integrated information system with primary functions that included the creative transformation of the medical risk-reduction messages into media events, the formative evaluation of those events, their distribution in coordinated packages over time, and their cumulative effectiveness in promoting change. The management of this system was put into operation by a process of continuous monitoring of the target audience's existing knowledge, beliefs, attitudes, risk-related behavior, and media use. The media campaign began 2 months after an initial survey and continued for 9 months in 1973; stopped during a second survey; continued for 9 more months in 1974; then continued on a very reduced basis in 1975 (Farquhar et al. 1977, Maccoby et al. 1977).

At the onset of the campaign, decisions were based primarily on data gathered at the initial survey, from the pretesting on local audiences of various media productions, and on the practical considerations arising from the likely availability of privately owned mass media. While the campaign was under way, further guidance was obtained from the second annual survey and from a series of systematic but informal small-scale information-gathering efforts designed to provide media planners with immediate feedback on the public's awareness and acceptance of specified sets of media events, as well as to gauge the progress to date. Thus, the total campaign could be seen as a set of phased media events where the information obtained from monitoring was used to refocus priorities, reset directions, and modulate the course of the campaign in the desired direction.

The intensive instruction program content was designed to guide the individual through tentative practice of the skills mentioned above, and gradually withdraw instructor participation. The expectation was that the behavior would be maintained in the group setting without the instructor. During the initial stage, intensive instruction was conducted in group classes and home counseling sessions. During the second year, the frequency and amount of contact was successively reduced. A less intensive educational campaign was conducted in the summer months of the third year.

The results of the education program, over a 2-year period, demonstrated a surprisingly large decrease in a composite risk score

5

for CVD. This risk score is an adaptation of one used in the Framingham longitudinal study (Farquhar et al. 1977). This decrease was about 25 percent for those exposed to only the mass-media campaign and about 30 percent for those who also received intensive instruction. The risk reduction in the community provided with mass media education was comprised almost equally of contributions from blood pressure reduction, blood cholesterol reduction, and decreased cigarette use. Among the individuals who received additional intensive instruction, a larger proportion of change was due to decreased cigarette use. Changes were reasonably well maintained during a third year of decreased education, especially for the intensively instructed group (Meyer et al. 1980; Williams et al. 1981).

Therefore, it appears that the amount of education provided, as described, was sufficient to produce impressively large decreases in predicted future risk of CVD in an adult population. The change when relying only on media education was especially surprising, given the generally poor results of prior media-based health campaigns (Robertson et al. 1974). Although no fixed standard of comparison is available, due to a combination of the difficulty in quantifying the amount of education and a general lack of well-evaluated health education studies, it does appear that, in areas of generally high public interest, a reasonably small amount of well-designed printed, television-based, and radio-based health education combined with a small amount of community organization and personal influence can produce substantial changes in knowledge, behavior, and physiological states that confer risk (Farquhar et al. 1977; Maccoby et al. 1977).

The experimental design involved development and application of a mass media and face-to-face instruction campaign. These communication efforts were designed to overcome deficiencies of previous unsuccessful campaigns to change behavior. Each campaign was intended to produce awareness of the probable causes of coronary disease and of the specific behaviors that may reduce risk. The campaigns also aimed at providing the knowledge and skills necessary to accomplish recommended behavior changes. Last, the campaigns were designed to help the individual become self-sufficient in maintaining new health habits and skills. Dietary habits recommended for all participants were those that, if followed, would lead to a reduced intake of saturated fat, cholesterol, salt, sugar, and alcohol. We also urged reduction in body weight through caloric reduction and increased physical activity. Cigarette smokers were educated on the need and methods for ceasing or at least reducing their daily rate of cigarette consumption.

For the mass media campaign, a coordinated set of messages was prepared for the audiences in Gilroy and Watsonville. Over time, these basic messages were transformed for a variety of media. The TCS demonstrated that mass media, when appropriately used, can increase knowledge and help people improve their health habits. The results led us to believe, however, that the power of this method could be enhanced considerably if we employed the media to stimulate and coordinate face-to-face instructional programs in natural community settings (e.g., schools, workplaces, community organizations). Thus, the TCS led to further investigation designed to test these ideas.

THE STANFORD FIVE CITY PROJECT (FCP)

The FCP began in 1978 and will continue until 1991 (Farquhar et al. 1985). The FCP differs from the TCS in that the two communities selected for education are much larger, the health education campaign is aimed at benefiting the entire population, the communities are more complex socially, the education program is more extensive, there are three reference cities rather than one, the education program will run for 6 years rather than 3, the effects of the intervention are being monitored for a wider age range (12 to 74), changes in CVD event rates (i.e., morbidity and mortality) are being measured, and a community organization program is being devised to create a cost-effective and lasting program of community health promotion.

There are two major hypotheses being tested in the FCP. The first hypothesis is that communitywide education can achieve a lasting reduction in the prevalence of CVD risk factors within a general population, leading to substantial decline in the Framingham multiple logistic measure of risk in a representative sample of persons age 12 to 74. The second hypothesis is that this risk decline will lead to a decline in CVD morbidity and mortality in persons age 30 to 74, and that this decline will be greater in the education cities than in the reference cities.

The education program of the FCP was introduced after completion of a baseline population survey. The effects of education on reducing risk factors are being assessed by comparing the results of the four independent sample surveys (cross-sectional) and cohort sample surveys (longitudinal) in the two treatment communities, with the results of the same survey types in two of the three reference communities. Epidemiologic surveillance of CVD morbidity and mortality is done in all five cities and will continue beyond the education program (Fortmann et al. 1986).

The education program has three goals. The first is to generate an increase in the knowledge and skills of individuals and in the educational practices of organizations, such as providing for exercise facilities and/or heart-healthy food choices and a smoke-free environment, to bring about risk factor reduction and decreased morbidity and mortality. A second goal is to carry out the education program so that a self-sustaining health promotion structure, embedded within the organizational fabric of the communities will continue to function after the project ends. The third goal is to derive a model for cost-effective community health promotion from the experiences and data accumulated in the TCS and this study that will have general applicability to other American communities.

The intervention itself consists of three components: broadcast media, print media, and community interpersonal programs.

Broadcast Media Components

The primary goal of using broadcast media in the FCP is to encourage lasting behavior change that will result in risk factor modification and, ultimately, reduction in morbidity and mortality. Underlining this major goal are two subgoals: encouraging direct behavior change and encouraging indirect change through support of community events. Some broadcast media products are hybrids: for example, a smoking cessation television show could encourage cessation as well as recruiting individuals to the smoking cessation programs available in the community. A wide variety of broadcast media programs are used, including public service announcements, TV news series, radio series and talk shows, and TV shows.

Print Media Programs

Print materials (e.g., newspapers, books, pamphlets, etc.) can usually provide more information than television and radio and therefore better skills training. Print media can provide messages of higher information density than can broadcast media, and they can be read and reread at the user's own pace, providing a large amount of information in user-oriented format. Reading print media can be greatly stimulated through the use of electronic media.

8

Print media products are distributed through direct mail and through existing organizations such as worksites and medical care providers. A variety of print media programs are used in the FCP. Big print is intended to carry a major message over a relatively long period of time. Media promotion print is any print piece whose primary objective is to motivate individuals to attend to the FCP's media events. Educational support print includes any pieces whose purpose is to support classes or workshops and includes reinforcing the knowledge and skills being taught in an educational program. The purpose of local print is to satisfy the projects' objectives of developing indigenous (i.e., community-owned) print materials.

Because of the large Spanish-speaking population in the intervention communities, mass media have included Spanish language. Radio production, for example, concentrates on Spanish language programs, since this is a major information source for this target group. In addition, weekly newspaper columns in both English and Spanish are a major part of the print media program.

Community Interpersonal Programs

The FCP community interpersonal programs are delivered through a variety of organizations, including health departments, community colleges, schools, voluntary organizations, health professionals, worksites, hospitals, and other nonprofit health service agencies. These programs include traditional strategies such as classes and lectures. They also include more innovative efforts such as incentive-based contests and use of lay leaders/role models.

Formative and Process Evaluation Methods

The program is being assessed by formative, process, and summative evaluation methods. There are at least seven specific topics in which formative evaluation assists in the design, development, production, and distribution of the educational program. These include:

(1)   audience needs analysis--understanding audience attitudes, beliefs, self-efficacy, and knowledge;

(2)   audience segmentation--identifying subsections of the community with factors in common such as needs, risk, demographic characteristics, and media use;

9

(3)   program design--addressing questions such as the proper name, location, and time for program and use of appropriate educational methods and materials;

(4)   program testing--testing an early version of an intervention with relevant audiences;

(5)   message design pretesting--to improve the effectiveness of specific mass media messages;

(6)   community event analysis--investigation of the factors that motivate participants to attend an event, how they learn about an event, what they thought about an event, and how this experience will influence their future participation and behavior change attempts; and

(7)   media event analysis--analysis of community media events.

A variety of process evaluation strategies are employed. It is essential to identify a number of steps in the process of community change and to measure each step. For example, while the ultimate outcome variable in these studies may be a change in morbidity and mortality due to heart disease and stroke, it is also important to measure intermediate stages such as success in community organization, knowledge, attitude change, skills learning, and performance and maintenance of these skills. One needs to know who changed in response to interventions. It is also important to evaluate the success of achieving stable and meaningful change in community practices and institutions as a measure of success in leaving behind a program that runs partly or totally on its own energies. While one cannot guarantee a totally clear explanation of success or failure, the use of process evaluation strategies will provide some important clues for future research and intervention.

Summative Evaluation Methods

The population surveys of health behavior on CVD risk factors are conducted by full-time FCP staff at permanent survey centers in four of the five cities. City directories of households, published by R.L. Polk, provide a relatively complete listing of households in each community (approximately 97 percent complete) and are revised every 2 years. All individuals 12 to 74 years of age who reside in randomly selected households at least 6 months of the year are eligible for the

10

surveys, are invited to participate, and are included in the denominator for calculation of participation rates (Farquhar et al. 1985).

There are two main types of samples included in the surveys: a cohort or longitudinal sample and an independent or cross-sectional sample. In the initial year of the survey, 625 people in each community visited the survey centers, comprising the first independent sample. These individuals were invited to participate in subsequent surveys every 2 years, to study the process of change in CVD risk and related behaviors over time. Second, third, and fourth independent samples will be selected over the last 6 years of the project to study cross-sections of the community without the potential confounding effects of repeated measurements.

The chief sources of data on health-related behaviors are questionnaires and dietary measures. The core questionnaire consists of the following components: demographic measures, attitude and opinion measures, health knowledge assessment related to prevention of heart disease and stroke, stress behavior, diet/nutrition and weight behavior, smoking behavior, physical activity behavior, communication media use and interpersonal communication network analysis, and medical history including medication use. Finally, a random 50 percent of the participants are given a 24-hour dietary recall, aided by food models to illustrate size, weight, or volume of foods.

A variety of physiologic measures are obtained, including weight, nonfasting venous samples (for lipid, lipoprotein, and plasma thiocyanate analysis), expired air carbon monoxide as a measure of cigarette use, blood pressure, urine samples (for urinary sodium, potassium, and creatinine measures), a low-level exercise test, and pulse rates.

Community Organization

It was always assumed that community organization would play a significant role in both the initial success and the durability of our program. In accord with this assumption, our educational program is conducted in a manner that encourages involvement from the outset by local community groups and is designed to lead to local ownership and control. Several assumptions underlie this approach.

(1)   Mass media education alone is powerful, but its effects may be augmented by community organization.

(2)   Interpersonal influence can be enhanced inexpensively through community organization, and this can allow a multiplier effect to occur that will increase behavior change.

(3)   Organizations can expand our educational program's delivery system in ways that are important for achieving communitywide health education.

(4)   Organizations can help the process of community adoption of risk reduction programs as their own, thus increasing the likelihood of continuing health education programs and maintained behavior change.

(5)   Formation of new organizations can be catalyzed by our external efforts to increase the array of groups concerned with health education and health promotion.

FCP Results

The results of the FCP are not yet complete. There will be a fifth independent sample and an additional cohort sample taken at the end of 1989. The surveillance of morbidity and mortality, which is expected to lag behind changes in risk, will be carried on for several more years.

Main interim results from the cohort sample indicate significant improvements in knowledge of CVD risk factors, reductions in blood pressure (both systolic and diastolic), and a reduction in pulse rate. Total risk, i.e., the multiple logistic function of CVD risk incorporating age, sex, plasma cholesterol, systolic blood pressure, relative weight, and smoking used as a predictor of a cardiovascular event within 12 years, was significantly lower in the cohort comparison.

Currently, the extension to self-help communities of programs of disease prevention and health promotion is being carried by the Kaiser Family Foundation with our staff serving as a resource center.

Summary of Community Studies

Findings indicate that the use of an interdisciplinary staff of cardiologists, epidemiologists, behavioral scientists, biostatisticians, and communication specialists makes it possible to mount community-based studies aimed at reducing the incidence and prevalence of chronic disease, especially cardiovascular disease. Methodologically, quasi-experimental designs involving the collection of a variety of demographic, physiological, and behavioral data can serve as baselines for prospective intervention studies and can assist in the design and creation of such interventions.

The TCS provided substantial indications that risk factors in CVD could be reduced through community education. The FCP is the attempt to replicate and extend these findings by additional means of intervention. Through these interventions, it is hoped that changes can be initiated and institutionalized with sufficient magnitude and duration to provide a means for reducing risk of, as well as morbidity and mortality due to, CVD.

THE STANFORD ADOLESCENT HEART HEALTH PROJECT

The Stanford Adolescent Heart Health Project is a 4-year, school-based research program conducted by investigators from the Stanford Center for Research in Disease Prevention. The project is designed to develop and test a multifactor cardiovascular risk reduction/prevention intervention for 15-year-old adolescents.

CVD begins early in life but might be prevented or delayed by primary prevention programs designed for children and adolescents (Berenson 1980). Interventions that only delay onset may still reduce the severity of the disease and the costs of medical care. Studies providing data on the effectiveness of multifactor programs designed to promote adolescent health behavior change in nonclinic settings are limited. Research is needed that develops procedures to help young people acquire and practice positive health behaviors and that measures the effects of treatment over time and with multiple indices of behavior change.

The Need for Early Intervention

Most researchers would agree that our modern lifestyle (cigarette smoking, diets rich in animal fat, sedentary habits) contributes to the development of CVD (Stamler 1980). Available evidence suggests that behaviors associated with cardiovascular risk are acquired early in life and may contribute to early onset of the disease (Berenson 1980; Stamler 1980; Coates et al. 1981; Lauer and Shekelle 1980). Autopsy studies on young soldiers (average age, 22) killed in the Korean war revealed gross coronary atherosclerosis in 77 percent of these men who had no known clinical evidence of coronary disease (Farquhar 1987). Elevated blood pressure, cigarette smoking, and sedentary lifestyle in college students have been shown to predict both fatal and nonfatal coronary heart disease (Paffenbarger et al. 1966; Thorne et al. 1968). Between 10 percent and 25 percent of adolescents are at least moderately overweight (Lauer et al. 1975). Sizeable numbers of children and adolescents show evidence of elevations in blood cholesterol (Lauer et al. 1975; Frerichs et al. 1976). Analyses of children's diets suggest that over 40 percent of the calories eaten are from fat in concordance with adult eating patterns. Saturated fat accounts for 15 percent to 18 percent of calories eaten, and dietary cholesterol is well in excess of 300 mg per day. It is well known that smoking rates among teenagers escalate sharply beginning in middle school and continue to rise into early adulthood (U.S. Office on Smoking and Health 1988). As Berenson (1980) has stated, "If today's children grow up like their parents, 20 to 30 percent of them will have hypertension as adults. Ninety percent will develop significant atherosclerotic lesions, and over 50 percent will die from hypertension and atherosclerosis." Thus, there is a clear need for preventive efforts beginning prior to the appearance of manifest clinical symptoms (Stamler 1980).

Advantage of a Multifactor Perspective

The Stanford Adolescent Heart Health Project is a natural outgrowth of earlier work conducted by Stanford Center researchers on the efficacy of school-based smoking prevention programs (Killen 1985). In this earlier work, senior high school students (aged 16 to 17) are trained to conduct smoking prevention programs in middle school (ages 12 to 13) settings. The high school students help to equip their younger peers with coping skills enabling them to resist social and cultural influences that promote cigarette smoking. This research has shown that prevention programs based on empirically tested social learning principles can help junior high school adolescents develop new health behaviors and maintain them, once training is complete.

The intervention was administered through physical education departments as part of the regular physical education curriculum. All 10th graders in each treatment school attended the experimental course sessions 3 days each week.

Health Behavior Change Programs for High-School-Aged Adolescents

Comparatively little health behavior change research has been conducted with adolescents 15 to 17 years of age. Successful smoking prevention programs and weight loss treatments developed for implementation in schools have been conducted in elementary and middle schools. While it is often assumed that interventions with younger children may prove more successful in achieving intervention goals, prevention programs may need to be delayed in order to coincide with developmental periods that favor skills acquisition and performance (Johnson 1982) or periods in which strong social influences to engage in unhealthful behavior occur. Thus, older adolescents may benefit more from treatment because they possess cognitive and behavioral competencies necessary to understand and act upon new health and behavior change information (Johnson 1982). One aim of this study (Killen et al. 1988) is to develop health behavior change strategies that take into account the influence processes specific to older adolescents.

Objectives

The Stanford Adolescent Heart Health Project includes the following objectives:

(1)   to collect data on the prevalence of cardiovascular risk factors in an adolescent population;

(2)   to develop procedures for building adolescents' self-regulatory skills and thus strengthen perceived competence in practicing healthy lifestyle behaviors;

(3)   to test methods for increasing adolescents' knowledge concerning the role of lifestyle behaviors in the development of cardiovascular disease;

(4)   to decrease the cardiovascular risk factor behaviors of cigarette smoking and excessive consumption of calories, saturated fats, cholesterol, and salt;

(5)   to increase the cardiovascular risk-reduction behaviors of aerobic exercise and complex carbohydrate consumption; and

(6)   to lower the risk factor variables of blood pressure and obesity.

Recruitment and Training of Teaching Staff

A 10-member teaching staff was recruited and trained to deliver the educational program. The basic classroom instruction was provided by eight full-time teachers. One additional staff person served as a coordinator and backup teacher in each of the treatment schools. The coordinator attended classroom sessions and had primary responsibility for monitoring the intervention to ensure that educational protocols were implemented correctly.

The core teaching staff was composed of young women and men in their early twenties, on staff with the Center for Research in Disease Prevention. All teachers had previous training in health studies and/or previous experience in health care/health research settings. A performance-based teacher training model was used to provide staff with the skills necessary for successful administration of the educational protocols. The educational program was divided into four basic modules. The teaching staff spent 3 days each week in the high school classrooms delivering the intervention. Teachers spent 1 day a week at Stanford preparing for the subsequent week's activities. During training sessions, teachers were first guided through the instructional protocols to acquaint them with the teaching objectives and strategies for particular modules. The staff then broke into smaller groups for rehearsal with feedback from group members. As a third step, teachers enacted protocols for the larger group.

Theoretical Perspectives Guiding the Intervention

If students are to adopt healthy lifestyles, treatment programs must build students' perceived value of acquiring heart-healthy behaviors; help them make immediate changes in current practices; help them generalize new practices to family, work, and recreational settings; and help them maintain new behaviors in the face of numerous personal and social inducements to return to old habits or to adopt less healthful habits.

The goals of the Stanford Project, based principally on Bandura's social learning principles (Bandura 1986), are to train adolescents with guided practice in which instructors first model appropriate counters to inducements to smoke and then help students to invent and use appropriate counters. The Stanford Project aims to provide strengthened environmental context for our intervention, because in a school-based program we are able to marshal environmental support necessary to sustain behavioral change. The environment may play a critical role in fostering maintenance by providing support and inducements for desired behaviors.

Education Components

The education program consists of 20 classroom sessions, each lasting 50 minutes. The 20 sessions are divided among five modules. Students in the education program receive an introductory module acquainting them with the concept of a healthy lifestyle and surveying the major risk factor variables: smoking, high blood pressure, and high blood cholesterol. This module discusses the benefits of weight control, physical activity, stress management, nonsmoking, and heart-healthy diet. A major goal of this module is to persuade students that various lifestyles may have important immediate effects on life quality as well as potential long-term health consequences, and thus to raise the incentive value of making lifestyle changes.

The emphasis on immediate consequences may be particularly critical or behavior change in this age group. Our surveys suggest that adolescent interest in health issues stems, primarily, from concerns for personal appearance and, to a lesser extent, physical conditioning. Therefore, dietary and physical activity changes may be accomplished most effectively by emphasizing relationships between health and personal appearance and condition. For example, dietary change may be most effective for some students when embedded in weight management programs.

A second goal of this module is to introduce students to the concept of self-regulation. This module demonstrates how self-regulatory skills may be used to achieve control over behavior. Specifically, students are shown how heart-healthy behavior change may be accomplished through the application of various self-regulatory techniques. Specific techniques include setting specific, proximal change goals, monitoring progress toward proximal goals, problem solving, use of self-instructional strategies, and applying self-managed incentive systems.

Following the introductory module, students are guided through a series of modules designed to provide them with detailed information on risk factor behaviors and opportunities to assess their lifestyle patterns. Thus, each module features information/demonstration and self-assessment.

As part of the final sessions devoted to problem-solving training, each student is required to carry out one self-change project designed to improve heart health. Special features of the treatment program include videodrama and role-play simulations.

Videodrama is designed to increase students' receptivity to altering risk factor behavior. Our previous work suggests that efforts to build appreciation for a heart-healthy lifestyle must precede behavioral skills training. As a first step in achieving this objective, a 39-minute videodrama presenting the contemporary, dramatic story of teenagers facing real-life situations and crises was developed. The dramatization was designed to increase adolescents' intentions to adopt and practice heart-healthy behaviors by producing a shift in their valuation of a heart-healthy lifestyle. Specific aims of the videodrama are to:

(1) strengthen students' beliefs in the positive benefits accompanying practice of heart-healthy behaviors (e.g., regular aerobic exercise);

(2) strengthen students' beliefs in the negative consequences associated with the practice of risky behaviors (e.g., cigarette smoking);

(3) reduce students' beliefs in the negative consequences associated with the practice of heart-healthy behaviors;

(4) reduce students' beliefs in the positive consequences associated with the practice of risky behaviors; and

(5) increase students' beliefs in their ability to assume personal control over their behavior.

Role-play simulations are designed to help students invent coping strategies for managing high-risk situations. Skill acquisition and performance are enhanced by rehearsal (Bandura 1986). Role-play simulations enable students to prepare themselves to manage difficult "real-life" situations and to devise and practice new behaviors under nonthreatening conditions. Behavioral practice serves an important role in the transfer of skills from school to home and recreational environments by boosting perceived competence in performance capability.

Evaluation

Measurements are obtained in school gymnasiums and cafeterias. Males and females are separated. Approximately 100 to 120 students are assessed during each 50-minute class period. Assessments consist of self-report questionnaires and physiologic measurements. Questionnaire and physiological data are collected for each classroom. Two days are required to collect data from all 10th graders in one school.

Two persons serve as monitors in each room. Monitors are trained to administer the questionnaire and to keep order in the classroom. Twenty measurement specialists are trained to collect the various physiologic data. The measurement staff are divided into specialist teams. Each team collects only one physiologic measure.

Preliminary findings suggest that the intervention has achieved a relatively strong effect (Killen et al. 1988). Knowledge gains in the treatment group are impressive. Changes in physical variables, particularly among females in the treatment group, may be indicative of the effectiveness of the intervention in promoting behavior change as well as increasing students' knowledge of CVD risk factor concepts.

Along with the analyses of CVD risk factor data, the research project has enabled us to make contributions in adolescent health areas outside our primary focus.

SUMMARY

Studies conducted by the Stanford Center for Research in Disease Prevention have been carried out over the last 15 years. These studies indicate that, with systematic planning by interdisciplinary research teams, field research projects, based on appropriate theory, can be mounted successfully both at the community level and in schools for the study of adolescents and for adolescent children.

Both final and interim results are for the most part encouraging. While all of the research reported here applies to health problems completely different from AIDS, some useful suggestions may emerge. For one thing, in both AIDS prevention and chronic disease prevention, the most effective measures to be taken appear to be behavioral. The research reported here is almost exclusively concerned with developing and testing methods for assisting people to change their behavior in ways that are likely to promote health and reduce risk of disease. They involve education at a community level and in schools. Perhaps education for AIDS prevention can follow similar lines with some success.

Recently, several studies have been directed toward the prevention of drug abuse habits being formed by schoolchildren. A 1984 Rand Corporation report summarizes a number of relevant studies and describes models that have been applied (Polich et al. 1984). These programs are aimed at nonuser adolescents who otherwise might become users. It depicts four stages of experimental use of drugs: (1) nonuse—never tried drugs, (2) experimental or episodic use, (3) regular or frequent use, and finally (4) heavy use. Primary prevention is aimed at the early stages of use. The methods used are essentially those described above. Students need to be able to identify pressures to begin usage, especially from peers. They then need to know the dangers and problems arising from drug use. Next, and crucially, they need to develop skills to resist such pressures and practice using the skills in the presence of such pressure. Role-play situations can help in this process. Project Star at the University of Southern California (not yet published) has recently completed a large-scale seventh grade study in Los Angeles junior high schools. They found the following social approaches worked best in the prevention of drug abuse behavior. These approaches promoted group identification, explained the nature of peer pressure, clarified the misinformation on the prevalence of drug use among peers, made clear the consequences of drug use, and used role-playing techniques to teach resistance skills. Results were assessed over a 3-year period and indicated success in delaying the onset of tobacco, marijuana, and alcohol use. They did not apply these methods to the prevention of hard drug use. Clearly such research is badly needed.

In research concerned with reduction of risk of CVD, the Stanford group elected to intervene at the level of the community for a number of reasons. Since risk of CVD is so widespread and since primary prevention was our goal, we sought to educate entire communities on the behavior needed for risk minimization.

It is also the case that communities offer a number of opportunities for such intervention. Organizations such as schools, media outlets, worksites, local health departments, churches, local health organizations such as chapters of the American Heart Association, American Lung Association, American Cancer Society, and many others offer means of diffusion that can multiply the education program's reach.

In this paper, such community studies have been described with a special emphasis on youth via schools. It is our hope that this model may have some applicability to problems of primary prevention of drug abuse.

REFERENCES

Bandura, A. *Social Foundations of Thought and Action*. Inglewood Cliffs, NJ: Prentice Hall, 1986. 497 pp.

Berenson, G.S. *Cardiovascular Risk Factors in Children*. New York: Oxford University Press, 1980. 453 pp.

Chaffee, S.H. Inter/Media: Interpersonal communication in a media world. In: Gumpert, G., and Cathcart, R., eds. *Mass Media and Interpersonal Channels: Competitive, Convergent or Complementary?* New York: Oxford University Press, 1982. pp. 57-77.

Coates, T.J.; Perry, C.; Killen, J.D.; et al. Primary prevention of cardiovascular disease in children and adolescents. In: Prokop, C.K., and Bradley, L.A., eds. *Medical Psychology Contributions to Behavioral Medicine*. New York: Academic Press, 1981. pp. 157-196.

Dawber, T.R. *The Framingham Study—The Epidemiology of Atherosclerotic Disease*. Cambridge, MA: Harvard University Press, 1980. 257 pp.

Farquhar, J.W. The community-based model of life style intervention trials. *Am J Epidemiol* 108:103-111, 1978.

Farquhar, J.W. *The American Way of Life Need Not Be Hazardous to Your Health*. Reading, MA: Addison-Wesley, 1987. 183 pp.

Farquhar, J.W.; Fortmann, S.P.; Maccoby, N.; et al. The Stanford Five-City Project: Design and methods. *Am J Epidemiol* 122(2):323-334, 1985.

Farquhar, J.W.; Maccoby, N.; Wood, P.D.; et al. Community education for cardiovascular health. *Lancet* 1:1192-1195, 1977.

Fortmann, S.P.; Haskell, W.L.; Williams, P.T.; et al. Community surveillance of cardiovascular diseases in the Stanford Five-City Project. *Am J Epidemiol* 123:656-669, 1986.

Frerichs, R.R.; Srinvasan, S.R.; Webber, L.S.; et al. Serum cholesterol and triglycerides in 3446 children from a biracial community: The Bogulusa heart study. *Circulation* 54:302-309, 1976.

Johnson, C.A. Untested and erroneous assumptions underlying anti-smoking programs. In: Coates, T.J.; Peterson, A.R.; and Perry, C., eds. *Promoting Adolescent Health*. New York: Academic Press, 1982. pp. 137-148.

Killen, J.D. Annotation: Prevention of adolescent tobacco smoking: The social pressure resistance training approach. *J Child Psychol Psychiatry* 26(1):7-15, 1985.

Killen, J.D.; Telch, M.J.; Robinson, T.N.; Maccoby, N.; Taylor, C.B.; and Farquhar, J.W. Cardiovascular disease risk reduction for tenth graders: A multiple factor school based approach. *JAMA* 260(12):1728-1733, 1988.

Lauer, R.M.; Connor, W.E.; Leaverton, P.E.; et al. Coronary heart disease risk factors in school children: The Muscatine Study. *J Pediatr* 86:697-706, 1975.

Lauer, R.M., and Shekelle, R.B. *Childhood Prevention of Atherosclerosis and Hypertension*. New York: Raven Press, 1980. 484 pp.

Maccoby, N., and Alexander, J. Reducing heart risk using the mass media comparing the effects on three communities. In: Munoz, R.F.; Snowden, L.R.; Kelley, J.G.; et al., eds. *Social and Psychological Research in Community Settings*. San Francisco: Jossey-Bass, 1979. pp. 69-100.

Maccoby, N.; Farquhar, J.W.; Wood, P.D.; et al. Reducing the risk of cardiovascular disease. *J Community Health* 3:100-114, 1977.

Meyer, A.J.; Maccoby, N.; Farquhar, J.W.; et al. The role of opinion leadership in a cardiovascular health education campaign. *Communication Yearbook* I. New Brunswick, NJ: Transaction, 1977. pp. 579-591.

Meyer A.J.; Nash, J.D.; McAlister, A.L.; et al. Skills training in a cardiovascular health education campaign. *J Consult Clin Psychol* 48(2):129-142, 1980.

Paffenbarger, R.S., Jr.; Notkin, J.; Kruger, D.E.; et al. Chronic disease in former college students 1. Early precursors of fatal coronary heart disease. *Am J Epidemiol* 83:314-328, 1966.

Polich, J.M.; Ellickson, P.L.; Rueter, P.; et al. *Strategies for Controlling Adolescent Drug Use*. Santa Monica, CA: Rand Corporation, 1984. 196 pp.

Robertson, L.S.; Kelley, A.B.; O'Neill, B.; et al. A controlled study of the effect of television messages on safety belt use. *Am J Public Health* 64:1071-1080, 1974.

Stamler, J. Their potential for the primary prevention of atherosclerosis and hypertension in children. In: Lauer, R.M., and Shekelle, R.B., eds. *Childhood Prevention of Atherosclerosis and Hypertension*. New York: Raven Press, 1980. 484 pp.

Thorne, M.C.; Wing, A.L.; Paffenbarger, R.S., Jr.; et al. Chronic disease in former college students. Early precursors of nonfatal coronary heart disease. *Am J Epidemiol* 87:520-529, 1968.

U.S. Office on Smoking and Health. Surgeon General's Report on the Health Consequences of Smoking: Nicotine and Addiction. 1988. 618 pp.

Williams, P.T.; Fortmann, S.P.; Farquhar, J.W.; et al. A comparison of statistical methods for evaluating risk factor changes in community-based studies: An example from the Stanford Three-Community Study. *J Chronic Dis* 34:565-571, 1981.

AUTHOR

Nathan Maccoby, Ph.D.
Stanford Center for Research on
    Disease Prevention
Stanford University
1000 Welch Road
Palo Alto, CA 94304

The Puerto Rican Intravenous Drug User

Yolanda Serrano

INTRODUCTION

Acquired immunodeficiency syndrome (AIDS) has come to represent one of the major afflictions of modern times, with tremendous individual and social costs. The groups suffering the most profound consequences of, and at greatest risk for, AIDS are ethnic minorities with the lowest national incomes, limited health care knowledge, and the poorest access to health care (Centers for Disease Control 1986; Bakeman et al. 1987). Historically, minorities have had limited access to quality care, primarily due to economic factors. Sociocultural barriers such as language, social class, education, and nonmainstream health-care beliefs have affected minority communities. A Puerto Rican who develops AIDS might suffer from already existing impaired health and might delay treatment until later in the progression of the disease. Based upon the experience of this writer, the result is that the number of persons with AIDS in the minority community is underestimated, and many more people of color are dying.

DRUG USE

Any examination of AIDS and the ethnic community must take drug use into consideration. The role of the addict is very important in the AIDS epidemic in three ways: the addict's contact with heterosexuals; the addict's use of needles, syringes, and other drug paraphernalia; and the risk of vertical transmission to the unborn child (Drucker 1987). AIDS is spreading at a faster rate in minority communities due to the progressive disease of addiction. Compounding the disease of addiction is human immunodeficiency virus (HIV) infection. Current estimates suggest that 1- to 1½-million people in the United States have been exposed to the AIDS virus (Department of Health and Human Services 1987). When citing

24

the extent to which intravenous drug users (IVDUs) contribute in the racial distribution of AIDS, the Centers for Disease Control (CDC) report that although Hispanics are 8 percent of the national population, they account for 14 percent of the U.S. AIDS cases (Centers for Disease Control 1986). In addition, Hispanic women account for 21 percent and children account for 22 percent of reported cases (Bakeman et al. 1987). The statistics concerning Hispanics and AIDS are grim. The Puerto Rican community in New York is unknowingly being devastated. According to the 1980 census, Hispanics comprise 19.9 percent of New York City's population, yet they represent 21 percent of the city's adult cases of AIDS. The New York City Department of Health indicates that 24 percent of all cases of AIDS were among Hispanics. Of the 2,765 Hispanic men with AIDS, 49 percent were IVDUs, 41 percent had sex with other men, and 6 percent engaged in both behaviors. For 4 percent, the risk category was unknown. Hispanics comprised 32 percent of adult female AIDS cases. Of the 474 adult Hispanic women with AIDS, 59 percent used IV drugs, and 30 percent had sex with a man at risk. Of the children with AIDS, 32 percent had Hispanic mothers (New York City Department of Health 1988a).

In Brooklyn, New York, which has a large Puerto Rican community, as of November 13, 1987, 274 (60 percent) of the total of 453 Hispanic males with AIDS were IV substance abusers; 133 (30 percent) were gay, and 21 (5 percent) were both gay and IVDUs. Of the 102 total Hispanic females with AIDS in Brooklyn, more than half (66 percent) were IVDUs (New York City Department of Health 1987).

The number of cases, particularly heterosexual and pediatric AIDS cases, is staggering. The infected IVDU transmits the virus to a sex partner, who then passes it on to the unborn child, changing the epidemic into a family disease in the Puerto Rican community. In the United States, the New York City area has the highest seroprevalence rate. The area also has the greatest number of AIDS cases among IVDUs. Over 75 percent of IV drug use AIDS cases in the United States have been from the States of New York and New Jersey. Blacks and Hispanics constitute 39 percent of U.S. AIDS cases, but 52 percent of New York City's AIDS cases (Des Jarlais 1987). In addition, New York has reported half of all the female AIDS cases in the United States. In New York City, which has reported over half of all the pediatric AIDS cases, approximately 80 percent of AIDS cases have been found in children of IVDUs. There are approximately 100,000 to 120,000 women in New York City of child-bearing age, and therefore contribute to more than 5,000 births per year. The majority of these women are Hispanic and black, who do not realize they are at risk or that their sexual partners currently use or have ever used IV drugs.

PUERTO RICAN DRUG ABUSER

In explaining the plight of the Puerto Rican addict, a better understanding of the economic conditions that have existed and are major factors in the incidence of drug use in the Puerto Rican community must be examined. The problem of IV drug abuse has disproportionately affected Puerto Ricans in New York. Therefore, IV drug abuse became a Puerto Rican problem. In a classic study of heroin addiction, Chein et al. (1964) reported a high correlation among high levels of drug abuse, low levels of education, and high levels of family breakdown in poor Hispanic areas. The same study found a relationship between those areas with fewer social and economic problems and low rates of drug abuse. The pressures of growing population, unemployment, poverty, overcrowding, massive displacement of Puerto Ricans from their neighborhoods, and continued dispersals in the city, combined with cultural and linguistic differences, have contributed to the disintegration of the Puerto Rican community. These factors place an enormous burden on the survival of the Puerto Rican family. The family is the heart of the Puerto Rican culture and the base of strength and support. The Puerto Rican addict's family is involved in most of his life, from growing up to courtship, when a man must speak to the woman's parents to declare his intentions.

Between 1980 and 1987, the Puerto Rican population in the United States grew by 35 percent, from 2 million to an estimated 2.7 million. According to the 1980 U.S. census 1,107,129; or 55 percent, were born in Puerto Rico and migrated to the mainland; 906,825, or 45 percent, were born in the mainland to Puerto Rican parents. In addition, about 43 percent of all Puerto Ricans in the United States (860,552) were living in New York City in 1980 (U.S. Department of Commerce 1980).

While the number of Puerto Ricans increases sharply, economic conditions worsen, relative to the rest of the Nation. Median family income for Puerto Ricans, as a percentage of total U.S. income, continues to decline. Whereas in 1959 the median family income for Puerto Ricans was 65 percent of white median family income, in 1980 it was 54 percent of total U.S. family income. In 1987, median family income was estimated at only 46 percent of all U.S. families.

26

Unemployment levels for all Puerto Ricans remained essentially unchanged throughout the decade as the highest among Hispanics—14 percent in 1986, compared to rates last year of 10.6 percent for all Hispanics, 5.5 percent for whites, and 12.8 percent for blacks. Approximately 42 percent of all Puerto Rican families in the United States are living below the poverty level. The urban tragedy that has occurred in New York City, the destruction of housing by burning, has contributed further to disorganization of families, along with the myriad of other problems.

The family is a traditional way of coping with difficult situations. If families are being torn apart by drugs, and there are no alternative ways to deal with the problem, then the future does not look good for Puerto Ricans. Puerto Rican addicts often speak of their families and their desire to go back to the way they once were. This is most apparent when entering a shooting gallery (places addicts go to inject drugs). When entering a shooting gallery, there is always a reminder of family life, with pictures, religious items, or other familiar objects. Poverty and joblessness place an enormous burden on the family's survival, family health, and family relations and contribute to the high incidence of drug abuse.

One way of attempting to reach the IVDU is by building bridges to their subculture (Des Jarlais et al. 1985; Des Jarlais et al. 1986). This contact can be achieved by culture brokers or outreach workers. Such persons have experience and training in both worlds. Through these informal networks, information can be transmitted to the IV drug abuser in a culturally familiar and nonthreatening environment. The culture brokers penetrate the addicts' social circles and promote behavior modification through frank and open discussion of HIV infection. These outreach workers also provide information regarding access to drug abuse treatment, medical services, and other social services. In dealing with addicts, experience has shown that they want treatment for their addiction, they are desperate to get off the drugs, and they always state they are tired of life on the streets.

WOMEN

AIDS is killing women. In New York City, HIV infection among IVDUs and their sexual partners continues to increase (New York City Department of Health 1988a). Many of these women are Puerto Rican. Addicted women are a special group. What has worked for other groups is not necessarily going to be effective for women. AIDS continues to affect women with the fewest resources, the women who are not ready to deal with AIDS. This population is at high risk for adolescent pregnancies. In New York City there are approximately 60,000 IV-drug-using women of childbearing age, according to the New York State Division of Substance Abuse Services. Women who are IVDUs have been victimized, traumatized, looked down upon, rejected by society and their own communities, and even rejected by their families. In addition, most people assume these women are prostitutes. These women are street addicts as well as women who use drugs secretly at home (housewives and students). There are also women in drug treatment programs who continue to inject cocaine. Many women engage in prostitution to support their drug habits.

An outreach program aimed at women and men in the sex industry must be implemented to provide AIDS education and referrals to health services and other agencies as needed. The program should be aware of and sensitive to issues affecting those working in the industry. Services should include referrals for general medical checkups, pap smears, breast examinations, sexually transmitted disease (STD) screening, full contraceptive services, pregnancy tests, drug and alcohol counseling, health and welfare information, free condoms, and other services. Literature for IV-drug-using women in the sex industry must be developed, with close attention paid to the Puerto Rican women. In view of the potential spread of AIDS, it would seem prudent to increase the level of understanding at street level as soon as possible. However, both prostitutes and their clients, predominantly heterosexual males who control the nature of the sexual contact and can transmit the virus to their families, must be educated. Present services are not geared to meet the needs of these groups. The greatest risks for contracting AIDS are multiple sexual contacts and sharing needles, syringes, and other drug para-phernalia. Therefore, prostitutes and IVDUs are major risk groups. In addition, clients of the prostitutes provide a pathway for the virus to enter the general community. Both groups are criminal and stigmatized and cannot be reached through regular channels. There is a substantial crossover between the two groups because a signifi-cant number of people belong to both groups. They share the same geographic locations and they are both exploited.

The problem's scope is easily demonstrated. If 1,000 prostitutes work in New York City (in the streets, brothels, parlors, escort services, or privately), and each has six clients per day, this adds up to 6,000 men per day. If each prostitute works 4 days per week (many work

7 days per week), then 24,000 men would have contact with a prostitute each week in New York City alone. These numbers are conservative. Through innovative and unique ways, IV-drug-using Puerto Rican women are being reached in New York City. Effective education on AIDS prevention and effective strategies for risk reduction must penetrate informal networks. Entry is made into shooting galleries, where women of all ages and all colors, pregnant women, women who have recently delivered, HIV-positive women, and women with AIDS-related complex (ARC) and AIDS are found. There are women living in abandoned buildings and shooting galleries, after becoming homeless when their sexual partners were incarcerated. The women who are living in the streets of Williamsburg, Brooklyn, the Lower East Side, Harlem, and the South Bronx are living a nightmare. Many are sick with abscesses, open lesions, syphilis, gonorrhea, and other STDs. Many are also pregnant and are not receiving prenatal care, since they do not have insurance.

Addicted women who become pregnant can transmit HIV to their unborn child. Most Hispanic children with AIDS are children of addicted Puerto Rican women or of Puerto Rican women are the sexual partners of IVDUs. IV-drug-using women and women in drug treatment programs rarely seek counseling about AIDS. They do not plan their pregnancies and do not participate in birth control. Many IV-drug-using women do not menstruate regularly. Their options are restricted when, at 4 months, they discover the pregnancy. Thus, early prenatal care is unlikely. Many Puerto Rican women have been turned away from drug treatment programs. In addition, many women become upset with the stringent protocol for admission to a drug treatment program. Addicted women also do not have a regular physician, and they rely on hospital emergency rooms for their medical care.

Clearly, there is a need to educate addicted women and women in the sex industry about the dangers of HIV infection. Women can be empowered to take control of their lives. Many women believe that if they are using a certain type of birth control (oral contraception), they are safe from HIV infection. The risk to Puerto Rican women needs to be more prominently placed in the literature and the media, emphasizing risk behavior and specific risk groups. Programs for Puerto Rican women must focus on enabling women to become more assertive in negotiating safer sex and condom use.

RELATED ILLNESS

A major concern for the Puerto Rican community is the dramatic increase in syphilis among men and women in urban areas, rising faster among black and Hispanic people. Nationwide, syphilis cases are up 35 percent this year over last year, with most of the increases in poorer areas of some major cities. The number of syphilis cases has more than doubled in New York City. There is a clear indication that the increase in syphilis among adults creates a rise in congenital syphilis among infants in poor inner-city neighborhoods (New York City Department of Health 1988b).

HIV infection is causing a resurgence of tuberculosis (TB) in New York City. This is evident due to the increase in TB cases among the sex and age group containing the majority of New York City AIDS patients (males 20 to 49 years of age). In recent years, TB cases in New York City have increased 36 percent, or 593 cases (from 1,630 to 2,223 cases), an increase greater than that for the Nation as a whole. TB increased 2 percent, or 513 cases (from 22,255 to 22,768) (New York City Department of Health 1988c; Stoneburner et al. 1987).

CRIMINAL JUSTICE CONTACT

The incidence of AIDS and AIDS-related conditions among Puerto Ricans and other ethnic groups who come in contact with the criminal justice system in the State of New York is increasing. In New York State, about 40,000 prisoners are incarcerated in State and city prisons. Blacks and Hispanics comprise 80 percent of the inmates, and Department of Correction officials have estimated that 70 percent of the State's inmates, or 28,000 persons, have a history of IV drug use (New York State Commission of Correction 1986). In New York State, 46 percent of inmates who have died of AIDS were Hispanics, 39 percent were black, and 15 percent were white. The Correctional Association of New York, which has legislative authority to inspect prisons, recently reported that inmates infected with HIV appear to have a very low survival rate.

OUTREACH TO PUERTO RICAN DRUG ABUSERS

Since 1985, the Association For Drug Abuse Prevention and Treatment, Inc. (ADAPT), an organization of recovering addicts and health treatment professionals, has gone directly into IV-drug-use neighborhoods and drug-injection sites (shooting galleries). Persons

30

from ADAPT describe HIV transmission and prevention and distribute sterilization kits. In attempting to change behavior among addicts, ADAPT has introduced three persons (facilitators) into the subculture of the IVDU in Brooklyn, New York. These facilitators are ex-addicts who are role models for active addicts and understand the risks and problems. It is hoped that one-on-one interventions can lead addicts to take steps toward self-protection and behavior modification.

A brief description of the facilitators' work may give an idea of their experiences. As the facilitators approach a particular city block, they begin to feel the mood of the block. Every block has its own mood, with a different population doing regular business and drug business. Each block is very well organized, with an army to guard and protect it. Lookouts signal the approach of any new person. A yell might be heard from one doorway to the next "todo esta bien," ("all is well") if the police are not in sight or a familiar face has entered the area. If a stranger enters the area, the word is spread not to do business with this unfamiliar person. Lookouts, also known as couriers and enforcers, will approach and threaten an unfamiliar person. Discipline is maintained by street violence. Pushers, dealers, and connections are all vital to the block's existence, as is the flow of drugs into the area. ADAPT facilitators have become known to addicts as people who sincerely wish to provide help. Facilitators are allowed access into the block and can stand near shooting galleries. They are also allowed to enter galleries, participate in private conversations, and, most important, facilitate behavior change. Behavioral changes observed by ADAPT facilitators include decreases in needle sharing and increased use of clean works. They also have observed addicts giving accurate risk reduction information to other IVDUs in shooting galleries or on the street. In addition, gallery owners have come to ADAPT members to obtain sterilization kits and referrals to drug treatment programs.

CONCLUSION

Minority communities, specifically Puerto Ricans, have been neglected. The result is that these communities are devastated by illness and death from HIV infection. There are hundreds of neighborhoods in which HIV is spreading at an alarming rate. A real danger is that HIV will become self-sustaining in the heterosexual community if we do not immediately provide the necessary resources to curb it. It is already too late for those with AIDS, those who are infected, and those children who will be born with AIDS. But it is not too late to stop further infection of Puerto Rican women who may become infected through their sexual partners. It is not too late to prevent further perinatal transmission to children. More weapons and resources are needed to fight AIDS and to avoid further casualties.

To reach IVDUs effectively, the problems of treatment cost and assuring fast treatment upon request must be addressed immediately. By bringing addicts into drug treatment, AIDS education can be offered and the process of behavior modification can begin. Treatment is prerequisite to behavior change. Addicts can change their behavior, and they care about their health and their families, but the disease of addiction is powerful. IV substance abusers and their sexual partners will need considerable help to reduce effectively the risks for contracting and transmitting HIV. To prevent AIDS within minorities, community resources for dealing with the many complex problems must be available. The family structure of minority communities must be utilized. There are particular strengths of black and Hispanic families that can be used to communicate information about behaviors that put IV drug users and their partners at risk for AIDS (Marin and Marin 1987; Triandis et al. 1984).

The IVDU is a member of several well-defined communities. Knowledge on how IV drug abusers relate to their culture and its structure and how these systems impact on IV drug use must be developed. Effective messages for Puerto Rican IVDUs, including the use of street jargon, must be developed. Community systems within each community, the family as a prevention/education network, and other relevant, culturally sensitive approaches can be utilized to reach the IV drug abuser.

The threat of AIDS to our society is very real. The writer of this paper has witnessed its devastation in minority communities. If you were to come into these war zones, you would see the virus at work and see its casualties. You would understand the urgency with which this paper was prepared.

REFERENCES

Bakeman, R.; McCray, E.; Lumb, J.R.; Jackson, R.E.; and Whitley, P.N. The incidence of AIDS among blacks and Hispanics. *J Med Assoc* 79(9):921-928, 1987.
Centers for Disease Control. Acquired immune deficiency syndrome (AIDS) among blacks and Hispanics, United States. *MMWR* 35:665-766, 1986.

Chein, I.; Gerard, D.L.; Lee, R.S.; and Rosenfeld, E. *The Road to H: Narcotics, Delinquincy and Social Policy.* New York: Basic Books, 1964.

Department of Health and Human Services. *Human Immunodeficiency Virus Infection in the United States: A Review of Current Knowledge and Plans for Expansion of HIV Surveillance Activities.* November 30, 1987.

Des Jarlais, D.C. Intravenous drug use and heterosexual transmission of HIV: Current Trends in New York City. *NY State J Med* 87(5):283-286, 1987.

Des Jarlais, D.C.; Friedman, S.R.; and Hopkins, W. Risk reduction for the acquired immunodeficiency syndrome among intravenous drug users. *Ann Intern Med* 103(5):755-759, 1985.

Des Jarlais, D.C.; Friedman, S.R.; and Strug, D. AIDS and needle sharing within the IV drug use subculture. In: Feldman, D., and Johnson, T., eds. *The Social Dimensions of AIDS: Methods and Theory III.* New York: Praeger, 1986.

Drucker, E. AIDS: The eleventh year. *NY State J Med* 87(5):255-257, 1987.

Marin, B., and Marin, G. Attitudes, expectancies and norms regarding AIDS among Hispanics. Presented at the Meeting of the American Psychological Association, New York, NY, August 1987.

New York City Department of Health. *AIDS Surveillance Update, AIDS Surveillance Division,* November 13, 1987.

New York City Department of Health. *AIDS Surveillance Unit Monthly Statistical Report.* February, 1988a.

New York City Department of Health. Remarks of Stephen Joseph, M.D. Comments of the Presentation to the Council of Black and Hispanic Caucus AIDS Briefing. March, 18, 1988b.

New York City Department of Health. *Tuberculosis and Acquired Immunodeficiency Syndrome in New York City: Special AIDS Issue #1.* March 1988c.

New York State Commission of Correction. *Acquired Immuno-deficiency Syndrome: A Demographic Profile of New York State Inmate Mortalities 1981-1985.* March 1986.

Stoneburner, R.L.; Des Jarlais, D.; Milberg, J.; Friedman, S.R.; and Sotheran, J.L. Evidence for a casual association between HIV infection and increasing tuberculosis incidence in New York City. Presented at the Third International Conference on Acquired Immunodeficiency Syndrome (AIDS), Washington, DC, June 1-5, 1987.

Triandis, H.C.; Marin, G.; Lisansky, J.; and Betancourt, H. Simpatia as a cultural script of Hispanics. *J Pers Soc Psychol* 47:1365-1375, 1984.

U.S. Department of Commerce Bureau of the Census. 1980 Census of
  Population and Housing, 1980.

AUTHOR

Yolanda Serrano, B.S.
ADAPT
85 Bergen Street
Brooklyn, NY 11201

AIDS Prevention for Non-Puerto Rican Hispanics

Barbara V. Marin

INTRODUCTION

This chapter develops a beginning framework for acquired immuno-deficiency syndrome (AIDS) prevention in Hispanic communities, which have not been as severely affected by the AIDS epidemic as the Puerto Rican community. This group, referred to as non-Puerto Rican Hispanics, includes Mexican-Americans, Cuban-Americans, and other Hispanics of Central and South American origin living in cities throughout the United States. It accounts for about 85 percent of the U.S. Hispanic population. While the epidemiology of the AIDS epidemic is very different for this group, many cultural issues, appropriate interventions, and research strategies will be similar for all Hispanic groups, including Puerto Ricans.

EPIDEMIOLOGY

At the present time, it is not clear to what extent non-Puerto Rican Hispanics are currently at risk of contracting AIDS. AIDS case incidence data indicate a lower prevalence of cases than the proportion of Hispanics in the population for all areas outside the Northeastern United States, except for males who are not intravenous drug users (IVDUs) (Bakeman et al. 1987). Because of the lag time between infection and illness, these case data suggest that human immunodeficiency virus (HIV) infections were occurring at higher than expected levels among homosexual non-Puerto Rican Hispanic men, but lower than expected levels in other subgroups of this population several years ago.

The limited data on current HIV infection rates suggest that the epidemic has now spread to non-Puerto Rican Hispanic IVDUs, although rates of infection do not approach those of Puerto Rican IVDUs. Studies of IVDUs in San Francisco (Chaisson et al. 1987) indicate that the proportion of Hispanics currently infected (14 percent) is far higher than the proportion of infected white non-Hispanics (6 percent) in the drug treatment and IVDU population. Although the potential exists for significant secondary spread of the virus through Hispanic bisexual men, IV drug use and secondary infections to nonusing partners and to fetuses are likely to be the major source of spread of the virus into the non-Puerto Rican Hispanic community.

CULTURAL FACTORS RELATED TO AIDS PREVENTION

Hispanic culture represents a particular set of values and norms that shape those reared in the culture (Hofstede 1980). The fundamental aspects of the Hispanic worldview are similar for individuals from different Latin American countries (Marin et al. 1987), even though many of the outward signs of culture (food, national holidays, dress) may be quite different. These cultural aspects must be studied carefully as they relate to AIDS prevention, to develop effective interventions. While these values are probably not easily changed, they must be respected and understood for interventions to be effective.

Familismo

One of the most important cultural characteristics of Hispanics is "familismo," or the emphasis on the family as the primary social unit and source of support (Marin and Triandis 1985; Sabogal et al. 1987). The strong family orientation of Hispanic culture creates a number of obligations as well as a source of perceived support in times of trouble. Hispanics feel a strong need to consult with other family members before making a decision, an obligation to help others in the family economically and emotionally, and a strong sense of love and nurturing toward their children.

Research on Hispanic smoking has revealed some of the power of familismo. Hispanics are far more likely than white non-Hispanics to express an intention to quit smoking because it sets a bad example for their children and might affect their children's health (Marin et al., manuscript under review). The power of a family-oriented message might also be used to combat AIDS. The impact of AIDS on the family and especially on the children could be a key motivating factor in prevention campaigns. At the same time, the value of children to Hispanics suggests that many Hispanic women will become pregnant and carry a pregnancy to term even after learning they are infected with the AIDS virus (Gross 1987).

Simpatia

"Simpatia" has no direct translation in English, but refers to the importance of smooth social relations. This is a central cultural value and social script (Triandis et al. 1984) that mandates politeness and respect and shuns assertiveness, direct negative responses, and criticism. AIDS prevention activities that involve confrontation, such as insisting on condom use with a sexual partner, seem inappropriate for this group. Polite and culturally appropriate ways to negotiate new sexual behaviors are needed for a Hispanic audience. The simpatia script also requires that the Hispanic listener appear to agree with a message, even though he or she has no intention of following the advice or did not understand it. This makes it crucial that intervenors ask questions to assure that AIDS information and behavior change messages have been correctly understood.

Another possible result of simpatia is that taboo topics are avoided in polite conversation. Given that both drug use and sexuality are taboo topics, these interventions will be more difficult.

Personalismo/Respeto

"Personalismo" refers to a preference by Hispanics for relationships with others in their social group, and "respeto" is the need for respect, especially for authority figures, in social relationships. These two concepts must be understood and put into practice for drug treatment and other prevention programs to be maximally effective. In practice, personalismo means that Hispanics may be more likely to trust and cooperate with health care workers whom they know personally, and with whom they have had pleasant conversations, often referred to as "la platica" by Mexican-Americans. The implication of respeto is that drug abuse treatment will be rejected if a Hispanic does not feel respected and valued. Another dimension of respeto is that often clients will not question an authority, even if they do not understand something that is said.

Although certain cultural attitudes common to Hispanics can hinder or support AIDS prevention efforts, many are amenable to attitude change efforts and intervention campaigns.

Sexuality

Sexuality appears to be even more intensely private and personal in Hispanic culture than in white non-Hispanic culture. Anecdotal information suggests that sexual issues often are not discussed even between sexual partners. Hispanic women may be very uncomfortable when a condom is presented to them (Compagnet 1987). In traditional Hispanic culture, the "good" woman is not supposed to know about sex, so it is inappropriate for her to bring up subjects like AIDS and condoms. Amaro (1988) found that married Hispanic women in Los Angeles had sexual relations infrequently and often perceived them as not particularly enjoyable. There is also a fairly strong double standard that allows men to have sex outside of marriage, commonly with prostitutes. Given the higher rates of HIV infection in Hispanic prostitutes found recently (Centers for Disease Control 1987), such a double standard is likely to result in additional spread of the virus. When asked about abstinence, some Hispanic men felt that not having sex would be nearly impossible as well as unhealthy for them (Marin and Marin 1987).

In addition to a general reluctance to discuss sexuality, Hispanic culture includes a fairly powerful homophobic component. One indication of this is that a nonpejorative Spanish equivalent for the word "gay" does not exist. Given this attitude, it is very common for Hispanic men who have sex with other men not to see themselves as homosexual, meaning that messages directed specifically at "homosexuals" or "gays" may be ignored by a large proportion of those at risk (Ronquillo 1987).

Machismo

"Machismo" is a complex phenomenon that may be both helpful and hurtful to an AIDS prevention campaign. The majority culture view of machismo as a negative, antifeminist phenomenon is not completely correct, since machismo has a positive dimension that could facilitate behavior change. Machismo incorporates the idea that the male has a serious responsibility to provide for and protect his family, an attitude that could be extended, by an AIDS prevention campaign, to include protecting the family from the threat of AIDS. A dimension of machismo that could create difficulties in AIDS prevention is the need for the appearance that the man is in charge. A Hispanic woman who challenges her partner because he won't use condoms, for example, may be setting herself up for rejection or possibly abuse (Gross 1987).

Promotion of condom use is likely to be difficult among Hispanic men who associate condoms with prostitutes. There is also a common belief that Hispanics will not use condoms because of the Catholic Church's prohibition against artificial contraception, but many Hispanics do use birth control (Potvin et al. 1968; Marin et al. 1981). Of course, whenever parishes or churches are the channel for AIDS prevention messages, condoms can be mentioned only in a very limited way (United States Catholic Conference 1987).

Other Cultural Attitudes

Some Hispanics in the United States, especially those who have recently arrived, use needles and syringes for activities other than drug use, such as piercing ears and giving injections of vitamin B12 and other medications (Compagnet 1987). This activity is partly due to the fact that in most Latin American countries prescription medicines (including injectables) are available over the counter. A recent study in San Francisco found about 5 percent of the Hispanic respondents occasionally injected medicines or vitamins in the home (Fairbank et al. 1987). There is at least one case of family vitamin injections spreading HIV infection (Koenig et al. 1986).

An assessment of information about AIDS transmission and prevention among adolescents revealed that Hispanic teens knew less than other groups (DiClemente et al. 1988). Some preliminary data suggest that many Hispanics view AIDS as a problem almost exclusively of the white homosexual community. When presented with the hypothetical situation that their partner had been infected with HIV, our San Francisco Hispanic sample often expected this situation to produce chaos, total abstinence, or abandonment (Marin and Marin 1987). Hispanic men seem especially likely to say they would abandon an infected partner, while women are more likely to say they would remain. These Hispanic respondents did not often make a rational, planning response to hypothetical news of an HIV infection in themselves or a partner (Marin and Marin 1987).

MODELS FOR SMOKING CESSATION AND PREVENTION AMONG HISPANICS

Community-level interventions are used to reduce a number of health risk behaviors, including cigarette smoking, alcohol use, and poor dietary habits. These community interventions provide information about the risk behaviors and how to change them, change community attitudes and norms concerning those behaviors, and ultimately affect the behavior of many individuals at high risk.

Currently, four large-scale intervention projects, funded by the National Cancer Institute, are aimed at smoking behavior in the Hispanic community. All of these projects are in progress, however, so conclusions cannot be drawn. Nonetheless, certain insights from these projects may be useful in developing an AIDS prevention campaign in the Hispanic community.

The A Su Salud/To Your Health project is attempting to intervene in two almost entirely Hispanic communities near the Mexican border. Behaviors attacked include smoking, alcohol and drug use, inappropriate diet and consumption of fatty foods, and not receiving regular medical checkups. This project is using a social learning approach in which role models from the community are presented via radio, TV, and newspapers, along with messages about how to carry out the behavior. In addition, lay counselors visit their neighbors to instruct and motivate them. Initial evaluations have indicated promising early trends (McAllister et al., submitted for publication).

A smoking prevention study in Boston/Hartford focuses on Puerto Rican adolescents. Change is being produced through community involvement, including production of videotapes used for discussion, contests, and school-based interventions. Anecdotal reports indicate that rap contests, which have also been used in San Francisco for AIDS prevention (Fullilove 1987), are quite popular among Puerto Rican youth (Carrillo, personal communication, 1987).

A Life Skills Training curriculum has been developed for drug use and smoking prevention specifically aimed at inner-city Hispanics. This school curriculum is based on earlier work with mostly suburban white adolescents; it teaches skills needed to resist peer pressure to engage in drug use, in addition to teaching general social skills (Botvin and Wills 1985). Preliminary results of the Hispanic curriculum are quite promising (Botvin, personal communication, 1987).

The Hispanic Smoking Cessation Research Project/Programa Latino Para Dejar de Fumar is a research project to develop and test interventions intended to help Hispanics quit smoking. Based in San Francisco, the project primarily serves Hispanics of Mexican and Central American origin. The objectives are to lower the prevalence of smoking in San Francisco Hispanics by (1) providing culturally appropriate information about the negative effects of smoking and the positive effects of quitting; (2) providing culturally acceptable techniques and services for quitting smoking; and (3) changing the community norms associated with smoking (Perez-Stable et al. 1987).

Pretesting of Interventions

Pretesting of all materials is essential to the development of effective AIDS prevention interventions. Development of Spanish-language printed or electronic media materials should be initiated by a bilingual-bicultural team.

One example of this process is the *Guide to Quit Smoking* developed and pretested for more than a year by the Hispanic Smoking Cessation Research Project. This process identified three general issues. First, writing simply and clearly is very important. A recent study of the reading level of 16 pieces of AIDS educational material revealed that the average reading level was grade 14, that is, second year of college (Hochhauser 1987). Such a reading level would be beyond the educational attainment of 80 percent of 18-to-24-year-olds and 74 percent of 25-to-34-year-olds (Hochhauser 1987). Thus, it is imperative that written materials contain simple messages, written at no more than fifth-grade level, which avoid regional variations in Spanish.

Second, pretesting should be used for format as well as for content. Our pretesting suggests that use of photographs of real people would be highly desirable. Reactions to the printed product have confirmed this—most people mention the beautiful photographs with Hispanic faces. Parents have reported reading the Guide to their children, which is almost certainly due to the large colorful photographs used. Those developing AIDS materials must pretest to determine whether testimonials, novellas, stories, family focus, scientific information, or some combination are most appropriate for their target audience. Given the importance of the family in Hispanic culture, some materials should be developed that could be used by the entire family.

Third, pretesting can enhance credibility. Some smoking cessation techniques in our research were quite acceptable for white non-Hispanics, yet were literally laughed at by our respondents. Others had to be modified to be more in tune with the culture. Rather than the "just say no" message used so often, respondents preferred to make up an excuse for why they were refusing a cigarette, even if the excuse was a lie. Saying no is rejected as too brusque and not "simpatico." It is likely that some common AIDS prevention messages will also encounter disbelief or seem inappropriate to Hispanics.

Multivariate Approach to Intervention

Anecdotal information from research with Hispanics as well as more formal research on other groups has indicated that behavior changes can be encouraged in large groups of people if health promotion campaigns use multiple channels to reach their audiences (Flay 1987). Mass-media-based attitude and behavior change has been shown to be effective, but high-frequency presentations and saturation are necessary for an effect. For AIDS prevention campaigns, a variety of channels can be considered including TV, radio, leaflets, billboards, posters, pamphlets, manuals, bus cards, hotlines, newspaper, community workers, volunteers, and community groups. These channels are discussed in more detail below.

To be most effective, a health promotion campaign must utilize the principles of social marketing (Frederiksen et al. 1984). In this approach, specific messages and interventions are aimed at specific subgroups in a community. In the case of AIDS prevention, specific interventions might be developed for teens, adult men, adult women, health care providers, Hispanic media, community leaders, persons at risk, and family or friends of those at risk.

AN AIDS PREVENTION MODEL

To prevent the spread of AIDS in the non-Puerto Rican Hispanic community there are two primary target audiences to consider: (1) IVDUs and their sexual partners, and (2) the community. The types of interventions appropriate for each will be discussed briefly below. Truly effective programs should include both of these components, since they will have a synergistic effect on each other.

When the principal target of prevention messages is the Hispanic IVDU, the types of interventions considered tend to be individualized and labor intensive. The objectives include decreased needle sharing, increased needle cleaning, and increased drug treatment, as well as safer sex practices. There are very little evaluation data on approaches designed to achieve these objectives among non-Puerto Rican Hispanics, but the potential approaches include: distribution and education about use of bleach, use of condoms, and needle exchange; provision of culturally appropriate drug treatment; and

42

education/counseling about AIDS for the IVDU and his or her sexual partner.

Along with individualized strategies, there is a need for more general, community-level prevention efforts. Such campaigns would be designed to create normative changes around AIDS prevention behaviors through multichannel, multitarget, culturally appropriate community efforts. Possible content, channels, and targets of such an intervention are discussed below.

The content of messages must be clear, behaviorally specific, and culturally appropriate. In the case of AIDS prevention campaigns, there are a multitude of possible informational, attitudinal, and behavioral messages, but many may prove to be confusing or offensive to Hispanics. Research is urgently needed in this area.

McKusick et al. (1985) identified certain prerequisites of AIDS prevention behavioral change. The individual must believe that AIDS is a dreadful disease, that he or she is personally at risk, that the recommended prevention behaviors are manageable, that he or she can actually perform those behaviors, and that the community and peers support this behavior change. While almost everyone believes that AIDS leads to death and there is no cure (Dawson et al. 1987), it is likely that far fewer people in the non-Puerto Rican Hispanic community see themselves as personally at risk, intend to carry out the prevention behaviors, or see others as encouraging those behaviors.

An effective AIDS prevention campaign must provide simple messages about a very complex subject. It has been suggested (Liskin et al. 1986) that the essential information to be transmitted should include: (1) those who are infected with HIV do not necessarily look different from anyone else or even know that they are infected, yet they are capable of transmitting the virus; (2) the virus is transmitted through needle sharing and intimate sexual activity; (3) the virus is not spread by casual contact (this may seem unnecessary, but persons who believe that it is spread casually are probably less likely to believe they can prevent spread); (4) women infected with the virus can transmit it to their unborn children during pregnancy; (5) a stable, faithful relationship with an uninfected partner is best, but, at the least, one should reduce the number of sexual partners; and (6) condoms offer good protection from the virus.

In addition, when the target group includes IVDUs and their sexual partners, it should be emphasized that a stable, faithful relationship is not protective if one's sexual partner is an IVDU.

Perhaps additional and somewhat controversial information might be added. Analysis by Hearst and Hulley (in press) indicates that the risk of infection from sexual intercourse with someone in a known risk group is substantial even if condoms are used, suggesting the wisdom of abstaining from sex with partners from known risk groups and partners whose sexual and drug use histories are unknown.

A community AIDS prevention campaign should request the active involvement of the community in helping to alert those at greatest risk. The majority of IVDUs live with at least one other family member (Cervantes et al. 1987), and some authors have called for a much more active involvement of the family in treatment (Sorensen and Bernal 1987). Marin and colleagues (manuscript under review) are currently attempting to identify which AIDS prevention behaviors Hispanic family members or friends would be willing to talk about with someone at risk and how they could broach the subject.

Community AIDS prevention intervention must utilize as many channels as possible, while tailoring messages for particular subgroups. Of course, some channels will be more appropriate than others for particular messages. Based on work with other community interventions for Hispanics as well as anecdotal information, it is possible to identify the following areas.

Radio and television are excellent channels for many messages to the Hispanic community. Radio is listened to almost as much as television is viewed, and most Spanish-language stations have popular talk shows that serve as good forums for providing information. Our experience with a 1-hour, once-a-month radio talk show about smoking has been very positive, especially when the format involved calls from the community. Television stations should also be quite cooperative, considering the positive reception of the program about AIDS produced in San Francisco, which included the videotape "Ojos que no ven" (Eyes that do not see).

AIDS prevention videos have the advantage of being relatively inexpensive to produce and useful in a variety of contexts. They can be used to promote group discussions. The greatest need is for Spanish-language information, but culturally sensitive English-language information is also needed, especially for adolescents.

44

Posted media include posters, bus cards, flyers, and billboards, and is certainly an often inexpensive way to achieve community saturation. We have been told that some of the most effective advertising of family planning services has been bus cards (Taplin, personal communication, 1987). San Francisco buses in Hispanic neighborhoods have bus cards that proclaim "Use Condones" (Use Condoms). These are simple messages in large print. However, in the Dominican Republic, a psychologist involved in a major anti-AIDS campaign reported that people were too embarrassed to read the posters (De Moya, personal communication, 1987). However, information and ads in newspapers were very helpful, because people could read them privately. Unless posted media have messages about AIDS that can be read quickly and easily from a distance, they may be ineffective in the Hispanic community.

Printed media such as pamphlets, brochures, booklets, or manuals can be printed and distributed widely. Articles and news releases should appear frequently in newspapers. Our experience has been that people in the Hispanic community tend to be quite unimpressed with pamphlets unless they are produced with full-color photos to attract attention.

Several cities in the United States and Latin America have Spanish-language hotlines for AIDS questions, which have had good success. And the NIDA-sponsored 800 number for drug referrals also has Spanish-language capability.

Word of mouth could be an essential channel for AIDS prevention messages. The most believable people for Hispanics are their own community leaders (Marin and Triandis 1985).

Physicians and other health care providers are also powerful sources of information in the Hispanic community. Few health providers ask patients about their sexual or drug use behavior (Lewis and Freeman 1987). This intervention, accompanied by written materials and referrals, may have powerful effects on Hispanics, given the great respect that physicians command.

There are a variety of other activities that might be considered for the Hispanic community, including AIDS prevention message contests, rap contests, production of videos or murals around AIDS themes, organizing neighborhood meetings about AIDS, taking materials about AIDS to friends and family members, talking to one's children about AIDS, volunteering for hotline service, or aiding and visiting persons with AIDS. One way that attitude change occurs is when individuals become personally involved in an issue and begin to speak and act on it (Bem 1972).

NEEDED RESEARCH

AIDS prevention research focused on non-Puerto Rican Hispanics is needed. In addition, difficult methodological issues must be addressed. Specific research needs include the following:

- Little is known about the sexual attitudes and behaviors of Hispanics, including frequency and types of prostitution, sexual practices and partners, sexual information given to children, or attitudes about sexuality and birth control. Accurate information about sexual practices may be very difficult to obtain, given the taboos surrounding this topic.

- Few studies have focused on Hispanic drug abuse. A bibliography of the literature available from the Spanish Speaking Mental Health Research Center (Hispanic Health and Mental Health Database 1987) revealed that the majority of studies have focused on the Puerto Rican population. Research is needed that is related to drug use attitudes, current drug use, needle use, needle sharing and cleaning, and the social context of drug use. Although the Hispanic Health and Nutrition Examination Survey collected information on drug use in the Cuban, Puerto Rican, and Mexican-American populations, these data currently are not widely available.

- Little is known about Hispanic attitudes toward AIDS and AIDS prevention, risk behaviors, normative pressures related to these behaviors, and cultural differences between Hispanics and other groups. Identifying the differences between those at risk who are able to change their behavior and those who are unable to change would be useful.

- Research is needed to identify the aspects of AIDS prevention that are culturally appropriate to Hispanics. This will include research on willingness to perform the various prevention behaviors, barriers to performance, perceived positive and negative consequences of these behaviors, and perceived approval of important others for these behaviors. Fishbein's Theory of Reasoned Action and Triandis' subjective culture approach should be helpful guides for such research (Ajzen and Fishbein 1980; Triandis 1972). Findings from Marin et al. (manuscript under review) revealed that important consequences of smoking and quitting were predicted by the research team beforehand (e.g., smoking is seen as a bad example to children); several others were surprising (e.g., cigarettes causing bad breath is a very powerful reason for Hispanics to quit).

- Culturally appropriate methods for recruiting and treating non-Puerto Rican Hispanic drug addicts must be developed and evaluated. Work with Hispanic families in this area might build on Sorensen and Bernal (1987) and Szapocznik et al. (1988).

- Culturally appropriate methods for preventing drug abuse must be developed and tested not only for those preteens and adolescents who are in school, but also for those who have dropped out. Approaches might build on the work of Santisteban and Szapocznik (1982).

- Culturally appropriate and effective programs to prevent delinquency, lower the rate of teen pregnancy, delay the onset of sexual activity, and prevent cigarette and alcohol use in adolescents should be evaluated. Problem behaviors appear in clusters and among friendship groups, so that effective programs addressing any one behavior will have an indirect impact on others (Jessor and Jessor 1977).

- The Association of Drug Abuse Prevention and Treatment (ADAPT) (Friedman et al. 1987) has been distributing bleach and AIDS education materials, and is attempting to set up a needle exchange experiment. Efforts such as these need vigorous evaluation to assist in future program planning.

- Community AIDS risk reduction programs designed to inform the community about AIDS, motivate the community to intervene with those at risk, and motivate high-risk individuals to change their behavior must be developed and tested. Specific questions to enable effective programs include:

  - Which AIDS reduction behaviors are community members willing to use themselves?

  - Which communication channels are most appropriate for AIDS prevention messages?

- What positive and negative consequences of AIDS prevention behaviors are most relevant to this population?

- Which persons are most likely to be able to influence the behavior of high-risk individuals?

- What is the social context of risky and safe behaviors?

METHODOLOGICAL ISSUES

In many cases, Hispanics cannot be identified, since only race is reported in some national and large regional studies (Dawson et al. 1987). To understand the epidemiology and prevention of AIDS, all large data sets, including the Centers for Disease Control AIDS case surveillance, epidemiological data on risk behaviors and HIV infections, and drug use and drug treatment statistics should be coded for Hispanic subgroup (i.e., Cuban, Mexican, Puerto Rican, Other). Future evaluations of community programs will depend in part on the availability of adequate archival data from these large data sets. Studies of research methods must begin to identify better methods of questioning Hispanics about sensitive subjects such as sexual behavior and drug use, so that data that are collected are correct and valid.

CONCLUSION

While AIDS cases among non-Puerto Rican Hispanic IVDUs are now low, a disastrous epidemic is possible in this group unless culturally appropriate prevention interventions are developed and evaluated. Current knowledge indicates that Hispanic cultural characteristics will have profound implications for interventions. These characteristics include familismo, respeto, simpatia, and personalismo, as well as sex- and drug-related attitudes and practices. Community-level prevention interventions must further identify culturally relevant beliefs and attitudes regarding AIDS prevention practices, as well as use a multimedia, multimessage, multitarget approach to saturate the community and change attitudes, norms, and behaviors regarding AIDS prevention. Research to identify the most appropriate intervention components is urgently needed. Many aspects of a program developed for non-Puerto Rican Hispanics may also prove effective for the Puerto Rican Hispanic population and vice versa.

REFERENCES

Ajzen, I., and Fishbein, M. *Understanding Attitudes and Predicting Social Behavior.* Englewood Cliffs, NJ: Prentice Hall, 1980. 278 pp.

Amaro, H. Women in the Mexican-American community: Religion, culture, and reproductive attitudes and experiences. *J Community Psychol* 16(1): 6-20, 1988.

Bakeman, R.; McCray, E.; Lumb, J.R.; Jackson, R.E.; and Whitley, P.N. The incidence of AIDS among blacks and Hispanics. *J Natl Med Assoc* 79(9): 921-928, 1987.

Bem, D.J. Self-perception theory. In: Berkowitz, L, ed. *Advances in Experimental Social Psychology.* New York: Academic Press, 1972. pp. 1-62.

Botvin, G. Personal communication, 1987.

Botvin, G.J., and Wills, T.A. Personal and social skills training: Cognitive-behavioral approaches to substance abuse prevention. In: Bell, C.S., and Battjes, R., eds. *Prevention Research: Deterring Drug Abuse Among Children and Adolescents.* National Institute on Drug Abuse Research Monograph 63. DHHS Pub. No. (ADM)87-1334. Washington, DC: Supt. of Docs., U.S. Govt. Print. Off., 1985. pp. 8-49.

Centers for Disease Control. Antibody to human immunodeficiency virus in female prostitutes. *MMWR* 36:157-161, 1987.

Cervantes, O.F.; Sorensen, J.L.; Wermuth, L.; Fernandez, L.; and Menicucci, L. *Family Ties of Drug Abusers.* Unpublished manuscript, 1987. Available from: J. Sorensen, Ward 92, SFGH, 1001 Potrero Avenue, San Francisco, CA 94110.

Chaisson, R.E.; Moss, A.R.; Onishi, R.; Osmond, D.; and Carlson, J.R. Human immunodeficiency virus infection in heterosexual intravenous drug users in San Francisco. *Am J Public Health* 77:169-172, 1987.

Compagnet, A. Hispanic culture redefines AIDS fight. *The Washington Post*, December 28, 1987. p. A1.

Dawson, D.A.; Cynamon, M.; and Fitti, J.E. *AIDS Knowledge and Attitudes. Provisional Data From the National Health Interview Survey: United States, 1987. NCHS Advancedata from Vital and Health Statistics.* No. 146, November 19, 1987. pp. 1-10.

DiClemente, R.J.; Boyer, B.C.; and Morales, E.S. Minorities and AIDS: Knowledge, attitudes, and misconceptions among black and Latino adolescents. *Am J Public Health* 78:55-57, 1988.

Fairbank, Bregman and Maullin, Inc. *Report on a Baseline Survey of AIDS Risk Behaviors and Attitudes in San Francisco's Latino Communities.* San Francisco: Fairbank, Bregman and Maullin, 5 Third Street, Suite 430, 1987. 99 pp.

Fishbein, M., and Ajzen, I. *Beliefs, Attitude, Intention and Behavior.* Reading, MA: Addison-Wesley, 1975. 571 pp.

Flay, B.R. Mass media and smoking cessation: A critical review. *Am J Public Health* 77(2):153-161, 1987.

Frederiksen, L.W.; Solomon, L.J.; and Brehony, K.A. *Marketing Health Behavior.* New York: Plenum, 1984. 200 pp.

Friedman, S.R.; Des Jarlais, D.C.; Sotheran, J.L.; Garber, J.; Cohen, H.; and Smith, D. AIDS and self-organization among intravenous drug users. *Int J Addict* 22(3):201-219, 1987.

Fullilove, M. Teens rap about sex. *MIRA Quarterly Newsletter,* 6025 Third Street, San Francisco. Spring: 1, 1987.

Gross, J. Bleak lives: Women carrying AIDS. *The New York Times,* August 27, 1987. Section 1, p. 1.

Hearst, N., and Hulley, S. Preventing the heterosexual spread of AIDS: Are we giving our patients the best advice? *JAMA* 259:2428-432, 1988.

Hispanic Health and Mental Health Database. *Drug Abuse/Drug Addiction/Substance Abuse.* Specialized bibliography No. 1. Los Angeles: University of California: Spanish Speaking Mental Health Research Center, 1987. 53 pp.

Hochhauser, M. Readability of AIDS Educational Material. Presented at the 95th Annual Convention of the American Psychological Association, New York City, August 1987.

Hofstede, G. *Culture's Consequences.* Beverly Hills: Sage, 1980. 475 pp.

Jessor, R., and Jessor, S.L. *Problem Behavior and Psychosocial Development.* New York: Academic Press, 1977.

Koenig, R.E.; Gautier, T.; and Levy, J. Unusual intrafamilial transmission of human immunodeficiency virus. *Lancet* 2(8507):627, 1986.

Lewis, C.E., and Freeman, H.E. The sexual history-taking and counseling practices of primary care physicians. *West J Med* 147:165-167, 1987.

Liskin, L.; Blackburn, R.; and Maier, H.J. AIDS - A public health crisis. *Popul Rep* [L]XIV (3):L-193-L-221, 1986.

Marin, B., and Marin, G. Attitudes, Expectancies and Norms Regarding AIDS Among Hispanics. Presented at the American Psychological Association, New York, New York, August 1987.

Marin, B.; Marin, G.; and Juarez, R. Talking to others about AIDS prevention: Preliminary analysis of cultural differences. Manuscript under review at *Health Ed Quarterly.*

Marin, B.; Marin, G.; and Padilla, A.M. *Attitudes and Practices of Low-Income Hispanic Contraceptors*. (Occasional paper No. 13). Los Angeles: University of California, Spanish Speaking Mental Health Research Center, 1981. 20 pp.

Marin, B.; Marin, G.; Otero-Sabogal, R.; Sabogal, F.; and Perez-Stable, E.J. Cultural differences in attitudes toward smoking: Developing messages using the theory of reasoned action. Manuscript under review at *J Applied Social Psych*.

Marin, G.; Marin, B.; Sabogal, F.; Otero-Sabogal, R.; and Perez-Stable, E. *Intracultural differences in values among Hispanics: The role of acculturation*. Technical Report #15. San Francisco: Hispanic Smoking Cessation Research Project, University of California, 1987. 31 pp.

Marin, G., and Triandis, H.C. Allocentrism as an important characteristic of the behavior of Latin Americans and Hispanics. In: R. Diaz-Guerrero, ed. *Cross-Cultural and National Studies*. Amsterdam: Elsevier, 1985. pp. 85-104.

McAllister, A.; Ramirez, A.; Amezcua, C.; and Stern, M. Experimental media and community: Programa A Su Salud. Submitted for publication, 1987 at *Bull of PAHO*.

McKusick, L.; Conant, M.; and Coates, T. The AIDS epidemic: A model for developing intervention strategies for reducing high risk behavior in gay men. *Sex Transm Dis* 12:229-234, 1985.

Perez-Stable, E.J.; Marin B.; and Marin, G. A smoking cessation intervention in Hispanics. National Cancer Institute grant 5 R18 CA 39260-03, 1987.

Potvin, R.; Westoff, C.F.; and Ryder, N.B. Factors affecting Catholic wives' conformity to their church magistirium's position on birth control. *Journal of Marriage and the Family* 30:263-272, 1968.

Ronquillo, Y. Prevention and Education in the Latino Community. Presented at the National AIDS Conference, San Francisco, November 4-7, 1987.

Sabogal, F.; Marin, G.; Otero-Sabogal, R.; Marin, B.; and Perez-Stable, E.J. Hispanic familism and acculturation. *Hispanic J Behav Sci* 9:397-412, 1987.

Santisteban, D., and Szapocznik, J. The Hispanic substance abuser: The search for prevention strategies. In: Becerra, R.M.; Karno, M.; and Escobar, J.I., eds. *Mental Health and Hispanic Americans: Clinical Perspectives*. New York: Grune & Stratton, 1982. 232 pp.

Sorensen, J.L., and Bernal, G. *A Family Like Yours: Breaking the Patterns of Drug Abuse*. San Francisco: Harper & Row, 1987. 194 pp.

Szapocznik, J.; Perez-Vidal, A.; Brickman, A.; Foote, F.; Santisteban, D.; Hervis, O.; and Kurtines, W. Engaging adolescent drug abusers and their families in treatment: A strategic structural systems approach. *J Consult Clin Psychol* 56(4):552-557, 1988.

Taplin, S. Personal communication, 1987.

Triandis, H.C. *The Analysis of Subjective Culture*. New York: Wiley, 1972. 383 pp.

Triandis, H.C.; Marin, G.; Lisansky, J.; and Betancourt, H. Simpatia as a cultural script of Hispanics. *J Pers Soc Psychol* 47:1365-1375, 1984.

United States Catholic Conference. *The Many Faces of AIDS.* Washington, DC: United States Catholic Conference, 1987. 30 pp.

ACKNOWLEDGMENTS

Gerardo Marin, Ph.D., and Eliseo J. Perez-Stable, M.D., provided critical review of an earlier draft of this manuscript.

This work was funded in part by U.S. Public Health Service grant DA 04928 from the National Institute on Drug Abuse.

AUTHOR

Barbara V. Marin, Ph.D.
Assistant Research Psychologist
University of California, San Francisco
400 Parnassus Avenue, Box 0320
San Francisco, CA 94143

Black Intravenous Drug Users: Prospects For Intervening in the Transmission of Human Immunodeficiency Virus Infection

Lawrence S. Brown, Jr.

INTRODUCTION

As we approach the closing decade of the 20th century, society finds a very formidable public health challenge with the acquired immunodeficiency syndrome (AIDS). As monumental as AIDS might be for the United States as a whole, its significance for black Americans is even more acute. While whites comprise the largest portion of the 53,069 currently reported AIDS cases (Centers for Disease Control 1988), blacks account for a larger portion of AIDS case reports than their percentage of the U.S. population. Indeed, although 12 percent of the U.S. population are black, 25 percent of all reported cases of AIDS are attributed to black Americans (U.S. Department of Commerce, Bureau of the Census 1980; Centers for Disease Control 1988). For blacks, the human immunodeficiency virus (HIV) epidemic could not have occurred with worse timing. AIDS adds insult to injury for a subpopulation of the United States already sustaining an excessive prevalence of illness and deaths due to cardio- and cerebrovascular diseases, cancer, diabetes, and chemical dependency (U.S. Department of Health and Human Services 1985). The human toll of the HIV epidemic among black Americans extends well in excess of the Centers for Disease Control (CDC) case reports of AIDS. While an indepth discussion of these issues is beyond the scope of this paper, it is imperative to make two crucial points. First, the face, or scope, of the HIV epidemic, even among black Americans, differs according to the prevalence of behavior patterns known to be associated with HIV transmission. Thus, significant geographic differences may and do exist in the prevalence of AIDS among blacks in the United States (Bakeman et al. 1986; Centers for Disease Control 1986).

Second, an equally important area of emphasis is that there are other medical, public health, social, and economic dimensions of the epidemic that often escape discussion. The concurrent rise in the prevalence of mycobacteria tuberculosis among black Americans (Centers for Disease Control 1987a; Centers for Disease Control 1987b) and the increased demand on already limited health care resources in many black communities are byproducts of the HIV epidemic. AIDS commonly claims the lives of individuals at ages most often associated with the highest levels of productivity to a society. For black Americans, who often reside in economically disenfranchised areas, the morbidity and mortality of HIV infection means further erosion in the economic base of these communities.

In the absence of an effective vaccine or a cure, education and prevention of behaviors associated with known routes of HIV transmission represent the greatest prospects for intervention. The success of these efforts has implications that extend beyond the medical consequences of HIV disease to the social and economic fabric of black communities across the Nation.

INTRAVENOUS DRUG USE AND AIDS AMONG BLACKS

A number of investigators have commented upon the association between various routes of HIV transmission and the overrepresentation of black Americans in the nationwide prevalence of AIDS (Hopkins 1987; Bakeman et al. 1987; Bakeman et al. 1986; Centers for Disease Control 1986; Brown et al., in press; Brown and Primm, in press). Although AIDS cases among black Americans have been distributed among the same transmission categories (homosexual/bisexual, intravenous drug abuser, heterosexual, etc.) as those AIDS cases occurring among the U.S. population as a whole, the tragic triad of intravenous (IV) drug use, belonging to the black race, and HIV disease is a recurrent theme in discussions of HIV infection in the United States. Epidemiological evidence demonstrates quite clearly that IV drug use occupies a prominent position in the prevalence of AIDS among women and children. The strength of this association is even more poignant for black Americans (Centers for Disease Control 1986; Brown and Primm 1988).

As demonstrated in table 1, black IV drug users (IVDUs) comprise an appreciable portion of the number of AIDS cases reported in the United States as a whole and in New York City in particular. Admittedly, the data in table 1 underrepresent the total contribution of injectable drug use because it does not include cases of AIDS that

54

TABLE 1. *Cumulative AIDS case reports among IVDUs and non-IVDUs in New York City and the United States*

	Total AIDS Cases		AIDS Cases Among Blacks	
	Non-IVDUs	IVDUs	Non-IVDUs	IVDUs
United States	44,025	9,044	8,746	4,664
New York City	8,739	3,997	2,143	1,835

have been associated with both IV drug use and homosexual/bisexual behaviors. Because the proportionate contribution of each transmission category and the racial/ethnic distribution of AIDS cases have been rather stable during the time periods displayed in table 1, a number of observations can be made. IV drug use alone is associated with 17 percent of all AIDS cases and 35 percent of black AIDS cases. Comparable figures for New York City are 31 percent and 46 percent. Viewed differently, AIDS cases among black IVDUs comprise 9 percent (or 4,664 of 53,069) and 14 percent (or 1,835 of 12,736) of AIDS cases in the United States and New York City, respectively (Centers for Disease Control 1988; New York City Department of Health 1988). The higher proportion of black IVDUs among AIDS cases in New York underscores a point made earlier in this discussion. The face of the HIV epidemic in the New York metropolitan area is largely influenced by the disproportionate prevalence of IVDUs in this geographic area (Brown and Primm 1988). Because the author is most familiar with the role of black IVDUs in the New York City HIV epidemic, the remaining discussion will focus on this population. Much of the information to be presented is derived from a number of seroepidemiologic surveys either published in the literature or from investigations conducted at the Addiction Research and Treatment Corporation (ARTC), a drug abuse treatment program that provides services to 2,100 patients in the boroughs of Brooklyn and Manhattan in New York City. In no way, however, is it implied that these findings can be extrapolated to all IVDUs or to all black IVDUs, whether in or outside of drug treatment.

BLACK IVDUS AND HIV SEROPREVALENCE STUDIES

Much of the information available on the rates of HIV infection in serosurveys are the results of investigations conducted of IVDUs in drug treatment. Very little seroprevalence information is available on the larger population of IVDUs not in treatment. Nonetheless, the expansion of HIV seroprevalence data among IVDUs has significantly increased knowledge of the prevalence of HIV infection. One fairly consistent finding across investigations has been the higher prevalence of HIV infection among black IVDUs as compared to their white counterparts (Chaisson et al. 1987; Weiss et al. 1985; Lange et al. 1987; Marmor et al. 1987; Friedman et al. 1987; Robert-Guroff et al. 1986). In 1987, among the HIV serosurveys conducted at ARTC (table 2), there was a trend toward higher prevalence of HIV infection among black IVDUs than for the entire IVDU population surveyed. This result was in contrast to results of surveys conducted in the previous years (1985 and 1986).

TABLE 2. *Trends in HIV seroepidemiology in ARTC for entire IVDU population surveyed*

Year	Number Tested		Seropositive	
	Total	Blacks	Total	Blacks
			(%)	(%)
1985	469	184	255 (54)	101 (55)
1986	262	100	159 (61)	62 (62)
1987	222	99	132 (59)	64 (65)

In reviewing the AIDS case-report data and seroprevalence studies among black IVDUs, a number of methodological issues must be considered. Particularly among seroprevalence investigations, closer scrutiny is important with regard to the geographic region in which these studies are conducted, the prevalence of drug use in these areas, the prevalence of various patterns of drug use and sexual behavior, and the laboratory screening and confirmation methods of HIV infection.

Admittedly, problems also exist in making reliable estimates of the number of IVDUs and the HIV infection rates among IVDUs. Regarding the former, advances in mathematical modeling are limited by the incompleteness of the system for identifying IVDUs. The prevalence of IV drug use is often estimated from information provided by law enforcement agencies and single State agencies having authority for drug treatment programs. It is important that the extent to which IV drug abuse has implications for exposure to and/or transmission of the HIV virus be clarified. While it might be inferred that IV drug abuse implies a high potential for HIV transmission, the impact on the HIV epidemic of those persons who infrequently use injectable drugs is arguable. Thus, in the context of the role of IVDUs in the HIV epidemic, information is limited by how we operationally define an IVDU and by restricted ability to determine the number of individuals who meet this operational definition in any geographic region. Conclusions about black IVDUs, like conclusions about IVDUs from other ethnic/racial groups, will be affected by this limitation. It is not immediately clear whether the effect will be to overestimate or underestimate the proportion to which black Americans participate in intravenous drug use. This problem also has significant implications for obtaining accurate information on the prevalence of HIV infection among black IVDUs.

TRENDS AMONG BLACK IVDUS

Having laid the background, inclusive of some methodological issues that affect research among black and nonblack IVDUs, questions remain concerning the extent to which ethnic/racial differences are associated with the prevalence of various HIV-exposing behaviors among IVDUs. It is obvious that this information would be invaluable to tailoring preventive efforts, should significant ethnic/racial differences exist. From the seroprevalence and ethnographic information collected in connection with the data shown in table 2, we find the following trends. Compared to the other ethnic/racial groups, black IVDUs tended to have a greater consumption of tobacco and alcohol, even in studies that controlled for age and duration of opiate use. The frequency of injection or sharing of needles/works by black IVDUs did not vary significantly from other ethnic/racial groups. In these studies, black IVDUs, compared to their nonblack counterparts, tended to have medical histories of a greater prevalence of clinical mycobacteria tuberculosis, a lesser prevalence of serum hepatitis, and an equal prevalence of endocarditis.

Because of the pivotal position of IVDUs in the heterosexual transmission of the HIV virus, ethnic/racial differences in the sexual behaviors of IVDUs is also significant. The practice of HIV-exposing sexual practices by IVDUs, in whom HIV infection rates are considerable, might explain why IVDUs serve as an important HIV transmission vehicle between the drug-abusing community and the general population. Ethnic/racial differences in the frequency of unsafe sexual behaviors, coupled with the ethnic/racial differences in HIV infection rates derived from seroprevalence data, might explain the overrepresentation by black Americans in AIDS case reports linked to heterosexual HIV transmission. While knowledge of HIV infection is limited, much less is known about the sexual behaviors of IVDUs.

From ARTC investigations, black IVDUs, in comparison to other ethnic/racial groups, reported a higher average number of sex partners and of sex partners with whom sex was exchanged for money or drugs. Compared to white IVDUs, black IVDUs also stated that a greater percentage of their sex partners were non-IVDUs. One sexual practice that has often been associated with HIV transmission is the performance of anal intercourse. The findings of the ARTC survey indicate that black IVDUs, in comparison to other IVDUs, either participated less in this sexual act or were less likely to admit to this activity. Interestingly, black IVDUs in our investigations were more likely to use condoms, compared to their white or Hispanic/Latino counterparts. Even the black IVDUs in these studies, however, admitted to using condoms for only 10 percent of their sexual encounters.

The literature (Eskola et al. 1978; Landmann et al. 1984; Glaser and Kiecolt-Glaser 1988), in describing a role of stress in modulating the immune system, stimulated our interest concerning the extent to which HIV infection was associated with the occurrence of stressful life events. One hypothesis is that stress-related events may place IVDUs at greater risk of HIV exposure and/or may sufficiently impair immunological responses, enhancing prospects for infection or the clinical consequences following infection. Alternatively, these stressful life events may represent other sequelae of HIV infection or disease. In the 1986 cohort described in table 2, we found statistically significant associations between HIV seropositivity and changes in employment status (p=.05), drug treatment enrollment (p=.05), and personal relationships (p=.004). Of particular interest was the finding that seropositive IVDUs were more likely to be depressed (p=.006) and lonely (p=.02). As far as black IVDUs are concerned, table 3 shows those variables where blacks, in comparison to nonblacks, experienced a greater occurrence of stressful events in their lives prior to enrollment in the seroprevalence study.

Perhaps the higher HIV seropositivity rates among black IVDUs observed in HIV seroprevalence studies might be associated with the greater occurrence of stressful life events. While the study design of the 1986 investigation did not allow for an assessment whether these events preceded HIV infection or were consequences of HIV infection, the role of stress in HIV exposure or progression deserves further study.

TABLE 3. *Stressful life events occurring more frequently among black IVDUs than nonblack IVDUs*

Event	Significance (p value)
Confrontation on Job	.041
Miscarriage or Stillborn Birth	.007
Losing Custody of Child	.043
Having to Get Welfare	.033
Child Got into Trouble	.047
Worrying Too Much	.045
Feeling Hopeless	.006
Loss of Sex Interest/Pleasure	.031

HEALTH PREVENTION EFFORTS AND BLACK IVDUS

Based upon the foregoing, AIDS-related interventions aimed at black IVDUs must effectively modify their sexual and drug-related behaviors. Stress reduction may also be beneficial in interventions targeted for black IVDUs. Unfortunately, there are many environmental factors that reduce the probability of reaching black IVDUs and positively modifying their behaviors. The environmental factors often associated with addiction promulgate its persistence and interfere with preventive behaviors. For example, a large body of data associates poverty with addiction. The communities in which black IVDUs reside are often the same impoverished ones in which their drug addiction began and in which effective preventive or intervention programs are not likely to exist.

Furthermore, the housing problem in New York City is a poignant example of how a response to homelessness can reinforce continued drug use. New York City's response of placing the homeless in shelters has resulted in many of these shelters becoming locations for the use or sale of injectable drugs. Because of the often degrading conditions of these facilities, many of the homeless commonly choose to stay "on the streets." In the experience of ARTC, the combined effect of the disproportionate number of blacks represented among the homeless and the large numbers of black IVDUs being homeless has significantly reduced the potential offered by housing and rehabilitating the drug addict. The rising prevalence of tuberculosis is also an indirect consequence of New York City's housing response.

Many municipal hospitals are experiencing a rise in tuberculosis admissions of patients with the following profile: black, IVDU, and occupant of a city shelter.

The response of many black community residents to black IVDUs can be characterized as either aggressively supporting law enforcement initiatives or passively encouraging continued sale or use of illicit substances. Primary prevention efforts in the public school system probably represent the most structured drug prevention programs in many black communities. However, the long-term effectiveness of these projects is unclear. School dropouts comprise the subpopulation that are less likely to receive these school-based efforts and more likely to engage in the illicit use of drugs.

Prominent in the black community is the church. On many occasions in the past, the black church has been a significant and highly visible force for social change. When it comes to HIV disease, however, the response of the black church has generally been silence and lack of support of prevention efforts. The clear absence of an affirmative/supportive response by the black church to the HIV epidemic is attributable to religious attitudes toward behaviors associated with HIV transmission. One such behavior is the use of illicit drugs. Some leaders of the black church have characterized the HIV epidemic as God's response to sinful behavior. The lack of support, underscored by such responses of black church leaders, represents another environmental obstacle to successful preventive efforts for black IVDUs.

With a notable exception, the preventive and health promotion efforts of many public health authorities often unintentionally exclude the participation of IVDUs. These efforts focus on facilities that IVDUs are unlikely to attend or at institutions with insufficient sensitivity to the problems of the drug addicted, white or black. From the experience of ARTC clients, hypertensive patients (an increasing number, given the rising mean age and overrepresentation of black patients) are not likely to have access to private practitioners or other nonemergency-room health care facilities for monitoring and followup of their hypertension. The absence of concern for the primary medical care of IVDUs by many single state drug agencies and the insufficient attention to the design of modest to large-scale health prevention efforts (thus unintentionally excluding IVDUs) by public health authorities has resulted in significant unmet health care needs among IVDUs. For black IVDUs, already living in economically impoverished communities with inadequate health care and human resources, this insufficient availability of drug-addiction-sensitive health care and social welfare services has been even more detrimental.

The notable exception referred to previously is in the area of prenatal services for IVDUs. Many large municipal hospitals in New York City have prenatal services specifically tailored for drug-addicted women. The facilities that are the most successful in reducing problems of noncompliance by the pregnant mother are those that have the following ingredients. First, the design of the clinics provides encouragement, education, and parenting skills particularly aimed at problems of the addicted woman and her often female-headed household. This does not mean just adding pregnant addicted women to a facility's otherwise established high-risk clinic, but providing sufficient, necessary, auxiliary services. Second, a close and intimate association has been established with the mother to reduce the inconvenience of having to attend separate locations for services.

Having reviewed a number of obstacles to prevention and health promotion efforts for black IVDUs, one may view these as monumental roadblocks. Nevertheless, these formidable challenges are not insurmountable. Innovative approaches and improvisation are the orders of the day. Important components of community-based interventions aimed at black IVDUs include: (1) the identification of the targeted behaviors and the provision of appropriately tailored HIV-risk-reduction education/information intervention by persons with sufficient rapport with black IVDUs, offered in locations with easy and frequent access to black IVDUs; (2) available services or vehicles to enable black IVDUs to translate acquired knowledge into immediate and sustained behavior change; and (3) the enhancement of traditional and innovative community institutions to provide support for positive modifications of the behaviors of black IVDUs. Finally, responsible program administrators of HIV risk reduction efforts must include systems for evaluating the effectiveness of their programs. Evaluating effectiveness will not be easy. In fact, in many ways the successful recruitment and retention of sufficient numbers of black IVDUs will mean a deemphasis on procedures or practices that attempt to identify the participants. The ability to truly determine the impact of HIV risk-reduction efforts targeted for IVDUs will require prospective studies with periodic behavior change assessments. Particularly among IVDUs, this will necessitate the collection of address and locator information for the IVDU and his family, close friends, and acquaintenances if loss-to-followup rates are to be minimized. These identification procedures are often seen by IVDUs as unwarranted invasions of privacy. Unfortunately, these same identification practices are key features of traditional evaluation methods. Thus, the challenge of caregivers for black IVDUs is to develop a range of innovative means to measure the effectiveness of their risk reduction programs. If black IVDUs are to receive the sustained support that they so desperately need, program administrators are going to have to meet the challenge of the vast majority of American society who demand evidence of accomplishment.

The scope of HIV risk reduction efforts for black IVDUs should range from primary prevention in school-based and nonschool-based youth programs to secondary and tertiary services (especially primary medical services) to be provided in drug treatment programs, public assistance/social service/child welfare centers, hospital emergency rooms, and the criminal justice system. While the latter locations provide points of access to black IVDUs, there is still a critical need for mobile vans and a cadre of "foot soldiers" to go into the shooting galleries and shelters where HIV exposure behaviors take place. The common theme is to bring the services (whether education, information, or primary medical or social services) to the black IVDUs. Furthermore, caregivers should provide a positive and supportive environment. Accordingly, continuous inservice training about drug addiction and its pivotal role in HIV disease needs to be provided to the service provider as part of the intervention.

As valuable as pure research is for mankind, research that effectively fuels community-based, risk reduction efforts for black IVDUs must be a high priority. There is a critical need to develop additional data bases to improve our capability to determine the number of IVDUs and to assess their primary medical and social service needs. Development is needed of mathematical models to use more appropriately the information substrate provided by various data bases. There is also a desperate need for research to assist program evaluation. Studies are crucial to determine what process and outcome measures (other than the diagnosis of AIDS/AIDS-related complex (ARC) or the use of HIV serological testing) are sufficient surrogates for HIV infection. Ingenuity is required to create instruments that assess behavior change and associated factors that influence behavior change. Creative ways to validate behavior modification are also in great demand. While it is ethically unjustifiable to postpone HIV risk reduction interventions until research efforts provide an acceptable volume of support in the foregoing areas, legitimate investigative efforts (for problem identification/monitoring, program direction, and evaluation) are critical if effective and sustained support is to be provided for black IVDUs. Research, appropriately directed, has the potential to be an important ally of caregivers in HIV-risk-reducing efforts. Indeed, research provides the evidence to inform a largely uninformed American public of the need to develop a more rational response to drug addiction and its medical-social sequelae.

CONCLUSION

For black Americans, the AIDS epidemic has meant a further insult to a previous state of excessive morbidity and mortality, a deteriorating family structure, and an impoverished economic base. While the face of the epidemic may vary in many geographic regions, IV drug use is a significant and pervasive factor in HIV disease among black hetero-sexual men, women, and children.

There are a number of formidable obstacles to effective intervention in IVDU-associated HIV transmission. Black community institutions, public health authorities, single state drug abuse agencies and gov-ernment agencies may all intentionally or unintentionally inhibit be-havior modification efforts directed at black IVDUs. Despite these environmental challenges, there are significant prospects for engend-ering community support, and there are multiple potential avenues to modify the behaviors of black IVDUs so as to reduce HIV exposure. The effect of numbers of current community-based outreach programs testify to this.

Significant demand persists for more education/information efforts and, more important, for health care and social services to halt the transmission of HIV infection and its sequelae. To be successful, future intervention efforts will need to be focused to follow two parallel, but closely related pathways. One pathway is to have drug abuse treatment mainstreamed into other health services. This will mean the modification of the curriculum of health professional schools and postgraduate training programs and modifying State licensing and professional certifying examinations to more greatly emphasize drug abuse and addiction. Admittedly, this is a long-term goal and would represent a true acceptance by modern medicine and society of drug abuse as a medical disease and a major public health problem.

The second pathway and more short-term approach is to diversify services within current programs of drug abuse treatment. Addiction to or abuse of one agent is becoming increasingly rare such that treatment facilities must have the capacity to respond to the

63

increasing prevalence of polydrug abuse. Many IVDUs admit to concurrent IV heroin and cocaine use. Additionally, many IVDUs are not likely to be accessed through traditional medical settings, necessitating that primary medical services become an integral component of drug abuse treatment programs. Funding mechanisms and drug treatment regulations should be reviewed and modified to encourage these program changes. While mainstreaming the drug abuse response is optimal, the reality is that the diversification of current treatment mechanisms is probably more achievable, although not a forgone conclusion. Public debate and political maneuvering may very well lessen the full potential benefits of either pathway.

Simultaneously, there is a need for further research on the identification and surveillance of HIV-exposing behaviors, on the validation of self-report instruments of behavior change, and on evaluation methods of current and future health promotion programs. Research is also especially needed to identify potential surrogates for sexually and parenterally transmitted HIV infection. Very little is known, for example, as to how well rates of other sexually transmitted diseases predict rates of sexual HIV transmission or how well hepatitis B infection rates are related to parenteral HIV infection rates. Presently, the opportunity for these concerted intervention and research efforts is great. Without these efforts, the price to be paid is too high.

Redefining the response to drug abuse for the American society is an opportunity that occupies a central position in the HIV epidemic. While taking advantage of this and other HIV-related opportunities is crucial for black Americans and black IVDUs, its public health significance is also great for the American society as a whole.

REFERENCES

Bakeman, R.; Lumb, J.R.; Jackson, R.E.; and Smith, D.W. AIDS risk-group profiles in whites and members of minority groups. *N Engl J Med* 315:191-192, 1986.

Bakeman, R.; McCray, E.; Lumb, J.R.; Jackson, R.E.; and Whitley, P.N. The incidence of AIDS among blacks and Hispanics. *J Natl Med Assoc* 79:921-928, 1987.

Brown, L.S.; Murphy, D.L.; and Primm, B.J. The acquired immuno-deficiency syndrome: Do drug dependence and ethnicity share a common pathway? In: Harris, L., ed. *Problems of Drug Dependence 1987. Proceedings of the 49th Annual Scientific Meeting, Committee on Problems of Drug Dependence.* National Institute on Drug Abuse Research Monograph 81. DHHS Pub. No. (ADM)88-1564. Washington, DC: Supt. of Docs., U.S. Govt. Print. Off., 1988. pp. 188-194.

Brown, L.S., and Primm, B.J. Intravenous drug abuse and AIDS in minorities. *AIDS and Public Policy* 3:5-15, 1988.

Centers for Disease Control. Acquired immunodeficiency syndrome (AIDS) among blacks and Hispanics--United States. *MMWR* 35:655-766, 1986.

Centers for Disease Control. Tuberculosis and acquired immuno-deficiency syndrome--New York. *MMWR* 36:785-795, 1987a.

Centers for Disease Control. Tuberculosis in minorities--United States. *MMWR* 36:77-80, 1987b.

Centers for Disease Control. AIDS weekly surveillance report. February 8, 1988.

Chaisson, R.E.; Moss, A.R.; Onishi, R.; Osmond, M.A.; and Carlson, J.R. Human immunodeficiency virus infection in heterosexual intravenous drug users in San Francisco. *Am J Public Health* 77:169-172, l987.

Eskola, J.; Ruuskanen, O.; Soppi, E.; Viljanen, M.K.; Jarvinen, M.; Toivonen, H.; and Kouvalainen, K. Effect of sport stress on lymphocyte transformation and antibody formation. *Clin Exp Immunol* 32:339-345, 1978.

Friedman, S.R.; Sotheran, J.L.; Abdul-Quader, A.; et al. The AIDS epidemic among blacks and Hispanics. *Milbank M Fund Q* 65 (Suppl 2):455-499, 1987.

Glaser, R., and Kiecott-Glaser, J. Stress-associated immune suppres-sion and acquired immune deficiency syndrome (AIDS). In: Bridge, T.P.; Mirsky, A.F.; and Goodwin, F.K., eds. *Psychological, Neuropsychiatric, and Substance Abuse Aspects of AIDS.* New York: Raven Press, 1988. pp. 203-215.

Hopkins, D.R. AIDS in minority populations in the United States. *Public Health Rep* 102:677-681, 1987.

Landmann, R.M.A.; Muller, F.B.; Perini, C.H.; Wesp, M.; Erne, P.; and Buhler, F.R. Changes of immunoregulatory cells induced by psychological and physical stress: Relationship to plasma catecholamines. *Clin Exp Immunol* 58:127-135, 1984.

Lange, W.R.; Snyder, F.R.; Lozovsky, D.; Kaistha, V.; Kaczanuk, M.A.; and Jaffe, J.H. HIV infection in Baltimore: Antibody seroprevalence rates among parenteral drug abusers and prostitutes. *Md Med J* 36:757-761, 1987.

Marmor, M.; Des Jarlais, D.C.; Cohen, H.; et al. Risk factors for infection with human immunodeficiency virus among intravenous drug abusers in New York City. *AIDS* 1:39-44, 1987.

New York City Department of Health. *AIDS Surveillance Update*. January 27, 1988. pp. 1-5.

Robert-Guroff, M.; Weiss, S.H.; Giron, J.A.; Jennings, A.M.; Ginzburg, H.M.; Margolis, I.B.; Blattner, W.A.; and Gallo, R.C. Prevalence of antibodies to HTLV-I, -II, and -III in intravenous drug abusers from an AIDS endemic region. *JAMA* 255:3133-3137, 1986.

U.S. Department of Commerce, Bureau of the Census. Vital Statistics, 1980.

U.S. Department of Health and Human Services. *Report of the Secretary's Task Force on Black and Minority Health*. Washington, DC: Supt. of Docs., U.S. Govt. Print. Off., 1985.

Weiss, S.H.; Ginzberg, H.M.; Goedert, J.J.; Biggar, R.J.; Mohica, B.A.; and Blattner, W.A. Risk of HTLV-III exposure and AIDS among parenteral drug abusers in New Jersey. The International Confer ence on the Acquired Immunodeficiency Syndrome. Philadelphia, PA, April 1985. (Abstracts)

ACKNOWLEDGMENTS

Drs. Robert Lange and Jerome Jaffe of the Addiction Research Center, National Institute on Drug Abuse, assisted by performing the HIV serological tests.

AUTHOR

Lawrence S. Brown, Jr., M.D., M.P.H.
Addiction Research and Treatment Corporation
22 Chapel Street
Brooklyn, NY 11201
                    and
Department of Medicine
Harlem Hospital Medical Center
College of Physicians and Surgeons
Columbia University
New York, NY 10037
                    and
Division of Health Administration
School of Public Health
Columbia University
New York, NY 10032

Community-Based AIDS Prevention Interventions: Special Issues of Women Intravenous Drug Users

Josette Mondanaro

INTRODUCTION

To date, women comprise 7 percent (3,653) of acquired immuno-deficiency syndrome (AIDS) cases (Centers for Disease Control 1988). However, the prevalence of AIDS among women is likely to increase, since the incidence of AIDS attributed to heterosexual contact is increasing. The Centers for Disease Control (CDC) estimates that another 7,300 to 36,000 women have AIDS-related complex (ARC) and that there are 50 to 80 times as many women who test positive for the human immunodeficiency virus (HIV) antibody as there are women with active cases of AIDS—at least 180,000.

According to figures from the CDC for 1988, women with AIDS come from the following risk groups:

Group	Number	Percent
Intravenous drug users	1,843	50
Heterosexual contact	1,074	29
Transfusion recipients	395	11
Undetermined	251	9

Although intravenous drug users (IVDUs) comprise the largest group of women at risk for AIDS, the sexual partners of IVDUs are the second largest group at risk. CDC figures show that, of women who were infected with AIDS as the result of heterosexual contact, 69 percent had their heterosexual contact with an IVDU and 16 percent with a bisexual man.

The fourth largest group of women with AIDS falls into the CDC category of "undetermined." It is believed that the women who fall into this category represent second-generation transmission; that is, their partners may not themselves be in high-risk groups, but may have had sex with others in a high-risk group. Many of the women in this group may be partners of men who are covering up their intravenous (IV) drug use, HIV-seropositive results, or sexual practices.

Thus, while it is difficult to estimate the numbers of women IVDUs, it is imperative to recognize that a successful AIDS prevention/ education effort must reach out aggressively to the following groups of women:

(1)   IVDUs in treatment;

(2)   IVDUs not in treatment;

(3)   Partners of IVDUs; and

(4)   Workers in the sex industry (prostitutes).

IVDUs Not in Treatment

It is estimated that for every chemically dependent person in treatment, there are seven who are not in treatment. Women, especially IVDUs, are underrepresented in traditional drug treatment programs.

Partners of IVDUs

It is reported that 80 percent of male IVDUs have their primary relationships with women who do not themselves use such drugs. As Des Jarlais and associates have reported (Des Jarlais et al. 1984), male IVDUs who become seropositive are typically not ready to disclose this information to their partners for fear of rejection and withdrawal of support. This coverup on the part of the male partners poses significant risk to women.

The nondrug-using female partners of male IVDUs may well constitute the largest "hidden" population of women at risk for AIDS. These women may not know that their male partners are IVDUs. They will be difficult to reach since they will not be associated with a treatment program.

Prostitutes

Women who work in the sex industry are at an increased risk of exposure to the AIDS virus based on a number of factors, including:

(1)   multiple sex partners;

(2)   anonymous sex with partners who may be seropositive or who may fall into one of the high-risk groups;

(3)   high-risk sexual activity;

(4)   IV drug use; and

(5)   decreased vigilance about proper safe sex practices because of their use of alcohol or drugs.

PROGRESSION FROM INFECTION TO DISEASE

Not everyone who is exposed to the AIDS virus will develop AIDS. In fact, researchers believe that the virulence of the AIDS virus depends on:

(1)   specific modes of transmission, i.e., direct intimate contact with bodily fluids;

(2)   repeated exposures over time; and

(3)   preexisting or concurrent conditions in the host (cofactors).

Unfortunately, many of the cofactors associated with AIDS are known to exist in drug users. These cofactors include poor nutrition, use of drugs known to suppress the immune system, repeated bouts of infection, and high stress.

Nutrition

Women heroin users frequently state that they use heroin to lose weight. Poor nutrition secondary to drug use is not just a by-product of poor eating habits, but actually results from the direct appetite suppressant effect of the drug. In addition, alcohol is known to exert a direct toxic effect on the gastrointestinal tract; this leads to an impaired absorption of food. Malnutrition is further exacerbated by inadequate assimilation of vitamins and amino acids due to damaged liver cells.

In some women, chemical dependency coexists with anorexia nervosa or bulimia. It is not uncommon for women with eating disorders to attempt to control their perceived weight problem through the combined use of drugs and starvation. Ultimately the body's immune system is compromised due to the chronic state of malnutrition.

Drugs

Drugs enhance an individual's risk for developing AIDS in multiple ways. Alcohol, nitrites (poppers), amphetamines, and marijuana are all known to suppress the body's immune system. Nitrites lead to a depletion of the helper T-cells by direct injury to these cells; they are also known as cofactors in the development of various forms of cancer.

In addition, the use of drugs to enhance sex may make it difficult to practice safe sex. Drugs which cause muscle relaxation and blood vessel dilation may enhance the absorption of the virus into the bloodstream. Decreased judgment and decreased pain sensitivity may make the participants less aware of the trauma involved in certain physical acts.

Repeated Bouts of Infection

Women drug users complain of medical problems more often than do men drug users. Indeed, it is often a medical complaint that precipitates a woman's entrance into drug treatment. Chemically dependent women are at increased risk for the following medical problems: infections, anemia, sexually transmitted diseases (STDs), hepatitis, hypertension, diabetes, urinary tract infections, gynecological problems, and dental disease, including abscesses.

During drug treatment, women continue to experience more medical problems than their male counterparts. While this may reflect a sociocultural bias (i.e., that women, more than men, are permitted to be medically ill), it may well also reflect the fact that drugs exert a more toxic influence on women. There is growing evidence that this is certainly the case for alcohol (Wilsnack and Beckman 1984). In particular, these drug-dependent women appear to be vulnerable to the traditional STDs of gonorrhea, trichomonas, and chlamydia, as well as the sequelae of exposure to these infections, which include pelvic inflammatory disease, chronic scarring of the fallopian tubes, decreased fertility, and increased abnormal cervical Pap tests. As a result of needle use or skin popping, IV-drug-using women also expose themselves to other infections, including abscesses, cellulitis, endocarditis, and hepatitis (Mondanaro 1981a; Mondanaro 1981b).

High Stress

Chemically dependent women experience extremely high levels of stress as compared with male drug users or nondrug-using women. Areas of increased stress include: responsibility for children, living alone, low income, low level of education, lack of financial resources, partners who are more likely to use drugs, more dysfunction and pathology in family of origin, higher levels of depression and anxiety, and lower levels of self-esteem (Reed 1981).

In addition, chemically dependent women tend to score high on recent life change events, which are other stressors.

PREVENTION MOTIVATION

Much of the AIDS prevention to date has occurred in the homosexual/ bisexual male community. These prevention efforts appear to have been highly successful. One prospective study reported that 80 percent of the respondents had substantially changed their sexual behavior from November 1982 to May 1984 (Coates 1985). Included in these changes are significant decreases in the following high-risk behaviors: numbers of new contacts, number of partners, receptive anal intercourse without condoms, oral-anal contact, and swallowing semen.

In addition, the number of rectal gonorrhea cases have declined by 75 percent in San Francisco since 1982. The San Francisco AIDS Foundation believes that this is a direct result of AIDS education.

Is it reasonable to expect similar prevention efforts to have such an equally positive effect on women who are chemically dependent? The response must be a resounding and pessimistic "No!" The demographics of the gay male population are diametrically opposed to the demographics of the female IV-drug-using group. One report of changes in sexual behavior of gay men in San Francisco studied 454 men with the following characteristics: some college (68 percent), white collar or professional work (77 percent), a mean reported income of $24,000 (Coates 1985). In comparison, studies of chemically dependent women demonstrate a level of unemployment that varies from 81 to 96 percent. Most chemically dependent women in federally funded treatment programs have not completed a high school education; even after completion of treatment, 72 percent of the women are still unemployed and lack the skills for gainful employment (Sutker 1981). Furthermore, AIDS statistics underscore the fact that ethnic minorities are overrepresented among women with AIDS (72 percent), as compared to homosexual men (25 percent) and all AIDS cases (39 percent). In fact, the cumulative incidence of AIDS in black and Hispanic women is more than 10 times that found in white women (Centers for Disease Control 1987a). These differences must be acknowledged and understood so that a prevention program can be developed that will be responsive to the unique needs of the chemically dependent woman.

EMPOWERING

To be effective, strategies for AIDS prevention and education for high-risk women must be based on empowering techniques. The process by which AIDS information is disseminated is as important as the content. The fear of contracting a fatal disease such as AIDS because of belonging to a high-risk group, coupled with the woman's sense of hopelessness and powerlessness, can be severely debilitating. Denying her vulnerability to AIDS or assuming the fatalistic attitude that she will contract the disease no matter what precautions she takes may be the woman's only defenses.

Chemically dependent women often feel like second-class citizens and are very sensitive to real or imagined messages that they are not worthy of help. It would be easy for such women to get the idea from AIDS prevention programs that they are being seen as unclean, potential spreaders of AIDS to more worthy members of society. It is important, therefore, to set any educational program about AIDS within the context of genuine concern for the well-being of the chemically dependent woman herself.

Didactic presentations will probably be the least effective method of reaching these women and bringing about both an increase in their knowledge and changes in their behaviors. Methods that involve these women in the development and delivery of their own programs are more likely to be successful. In every client and community population, there are individuals who are highly respected and recognized by other members of that identified group and make up an informal network of indigenous community helpers. These individuals can become an integral part of the community's educational efforts by bridging the gap between the formal organizations and the various populations of high-risk women.

The techniques of activating clients and identifying natural helpers can be utilized within the drug treatment programs, in jail and prison settings, with groups of women who work in the sex industry, and within the community at large. Information given by these trusted individuals will carry more weight than information given by drug treatment counselors, jail guards, or other people who may not be perceived as having the woman's well-being as their primary goal. Natural helpers can be identified and selected from all the groups of women that a program wishes to reach. Depending on the location and situation, target groups may be broken down by drugs of choice (i.e., IV speed users, IV heroin users), ethnicity, area of residence, or any other grouping.

Formal drug programs and other community organizations can offer space for meetings, printed educational material, resource lists, and other tangible support for the informal networking being carried out by the natural helpers.

"Coyote," the national organization for women in the sex industry, has written its own guidelines for AIDS prevention. In addition, it holds open meetings called The Bad Girls Rap Group, during which women can discuss their concerns and have their questions answered in a supportive, nonthreatening environment. This type of organizing builds on the strengths found in a particular group. For example, women who work in the sex industry often practice safe sex and are very knowledgeable about techniques for avoiding STDs. These skills can be acknowledged and used to teach women who may not be quite as familiar with safe sex practices.

It is imperative that programs assist women in taking control of their own lives. It should be remembered that the process by which a program reaches women will make the difference between success and failure.

EDUCATION AND OUTREACH

Education and outreach to prevent the transmission of AIDS will require a multilevel approach, involving a variety of organizations that provide services to women. Women at risk can be reached through the following agencies: public health departments, family planning clinics, social service agencies, city and county jails, State prisons, women's health centers, battered women's shelters, women's crisis programs, and drug treatment programs.

Service agency staff and members of the at-risk groups should be trained to give the training themselves (Mondanaro et al. 1982). Specific strategies that have been used to reach women include: outreach to health providers, development of an advocacy and information network of women working on AIDS issues, direct media advertising, use of existing community institutions including health, social service, ethnic, religious, and other cultural organizations, material development in appropriate languages incorporating AIDS information into existing materials, and hotlines, mass-media education, and multiethnic outreach (Shaw 1985).

Areas to be covered by any intervention approach used with women should include safe sex practices, changing sexual behaviors, and pregnancy.

Safe and Unsafe Sex Practices

In this culture, there are very few words with which to adequately discuss sex and bodily parts. Vocabulary is limited to scientific medical jargon, street-wise "dirty" words, or baby talk. It is important that the words selected are understood by all and that street talk not be avoided because of the discomfort of the educator. At the same time, a sense of respect and dignity must be communicated while using common terms. Most persons are often uncomfortable in dealing with issues of sexuality, and specialized training should be offered to prepare intervention staff properly.

Safe sex includes activities that involve only skin-to-skin contact, where there are no breaks in the skin from sores, infections, or wounds. These activities include: massages, hugging, body-to-body rubbing, social (dry) kissing, voyeurism, exhibitionism, fantasy, touching one's own genitals, and using one's own sex toys.

Using condoms, latex gloves, and latex barriers to avoid exchanging bodily fluids--semen, saliva, urine, feces, or blood--is safe as long as they are used properly and do not come off or break. The proper use of these protective devices will allow a couple to engage safely in vaginal intercourse (with a condom), fellatio (with a condom), cunnilingus (with a latex barrier), and hand/finger-to-genital contact (with latex gloves).

Changing Sexual Behaviors

Practicing safe sex may pose a substantial challenge for chemically dependent women. These women are being asked to change both their drug-taking behaviors and their sexual behaviors. Many chemically dependent women already experience difficulty in the area of sexuality. For some women, sexuality is the only way they know to experience intimacy. Intervention programs must appreciate the core changes that are being demanded of these women. In addition, women may be afraid to tell their partners that they need to change their sexual practices. They may fear rejection and abandonment, and their fears may not be unwarranted.

Despite a hardened exterior, these women are often exceptionally passive as a result of strict sex-role socialization; they have learned that to be feminine means to be passive and nonassertive. These women often test at the extreme end of feminine, while their chemically dependent male partners test at the extreme end of masculine (Mondanaro et al. 1982). The result is that the woman may be too passive to exert herself and the man may not accept his responsibility or cooperate in sexual risk reduction. The male partner may see changes in sexual practices as unmasculine.

Intervention programs must assist chemically dependent women to escape from this socially passive role. Women role models will be extremely important in getting across the message that a woman must take responsibility for her own body. Natural helpers can be of great assistance in modeling assertive behavior and in giving the women permission to do things differently.

Anticipating a woman's hesitation and discomfort, providing support, and creating opportunities for role playing will all help increase her confidence. Warnings about AIDS could be misinterpreted to mean that these women are not to have any fun or pleasure in their lives. Frank discussion should take place about how to enjoy sex and keep it safe at the same time. These sessions will be more believable if presented by individuals who truly believe that safe sex can be fully satisfying and enjoyable.

It is imperative that all women who are IVDUs, partners of IVDUs, or prostitutes, or who have sex with anonymous or multiple partners practice safe sex. Material regarding testing and seropositivity may confuse the basic, simple message that all women in these high-risk groups must practice safe sex.

76

Pregnancy and AIDS

According to the CDC, 80 percent of pediatric AIDS cases are attributed to transmission from an infected parent (Centers for Disease Control 1987b). In 90 percent of these cases, the babies' mothers either used drugs intravenously or had male sexual partners who used IV drugs. Ethnic minority children comprise 80 percent of all pediatric AIDS cases (Centers for Disease Control 1986). The bulk of these cases represent *in utero* transmission. Another potential source for contracting the virus is artificial insemination. Lesbians and other women who received donor semen are being followed in a San Francisco study to see if they have developed antibodies to HIV.

Chemically dependent women have been told that they should be tested for HIV prior to pregnancy. This is good advice, but ignores the reality that most pregnant addicts have not planned their pregnancies. Amenorrhea, a result of heroin use, or decreased fertility as a result of repeated bouts of pelvic inflammatory disease make some chemically dependent women believe that they cannot get pregnant. Other women are too preoccupied with drugs to even think about the possibility or need for contraception.

Contraception information must be made a major component of any AIDS prevention/education program for women. This should include the evaluation of women who falsely believe that they cannot get pregnant because they have scarring secondary to infections in the fallopian tubes. These women may have diminished fertility because of heroin use, but once they enter treatment and become abstinent from heroin, their fertility increases.

Pregnancy is associated with suppression of immunity, particularly cell-mediated immunity. This is especially true during the last 3 months of pregnancy and is evident up to 3 months after delivery. It is known that this decreased immunity increases a woman's susceptibility to certain infections, and it is believed that it can make a pregnant woman more vulnerable to developing AIDS, especially if she is already seropositive (Centers for Disease Control 1985).

INFORMATION THAT ALL WOMEN SHOULD KNOW

There is some information that should be given to all women in high-risk groups, regardless of their HIV antibody status. The basic information about AIDS should include:

(1)   a fundamental description of AIDS;

(2)   the iceberg concept, which explains that AIDS represents only
        the end of a continuum that also includes HIV seropositivity and
        ARC;

(3)   the fact that healthy people can be carriers of AIDS and that
        whether an IVDU is contagious for AIDS cannot be told by
        his/her physical appearance;

(4)   how they can become infected, i.e., IV drug use, sharing of
        needles, sex with IVDUs, sex with a man whose history is
        unknown, and sex with multiple sex partners; and

(5)   AIDS is not spread by casual contact.

What women should know about pregnancy and AIDS includes:

(1)   73 percent of pediatric AIDS is attributed to maternal transmis-
        sion during pregnancy;

(2)   a seropositive woman does not need to be sick with the disease
        of AIDS to pass the disease on to her fetus;

(3)   50 to 60 percent of children born to seropositive mothers will
        be infected;

(4)   there is no way to prevent the fetus from becoming
        infected if the mother is infected;

(5)   infants and children of seropositive mothers must be carefully
        monitored because the infection may not cause symptoms
        immediately at birth;

(6)   pregnancy is a stress on the woman's body and as such may
        increase the chances of an infected woman developing
        symptoms;

(7)   seropositive women should not get pregnant;

(8)   high-risk women should get an HIV antibody test prior to get-
        ting pregnant;

(9)   the virus is passed in the breast milk, and seropositive women should avoid breast feeding; and

(10)   women in high-risk groups who do become pregnant should get the HIV antibody test.

Women who are seropositive, but have no symptoms, should be told that regular medical evaluations and followup are advised. They are probably both infected for life and contagious for life and must act as if they are contagious. They cannot assume they will or will not develop AIDS. Any persons who have been exposed to the seropositive woman, i.e., sexual partners, children, and persons with whom needles have been shared, should seek HIV testing. It is still true that repeated exposures to the virus may increase the chances of developing AIDS; therefore, they should not have unsafe sex or share needles with other seropositive individuals. Meanwhile, maintenance efforts, including proper nutrition, abstinence and sobriety, stress management, safe sex practices, and no sharing of needles may all decrease the risk of seropositivity developing into ARC or AIDS. They should not get pregnant and should use a reliable method of birth control. Of course, they should not donate blood, plasma, body organs, or other tissue. Further, when seeking medical or dental care, they should inform health care providers of their positive antibody status, so that appropriate care can be given and precautions taken to prevent transmission.

The seropositive woman can be assured that the virus is not spread through casual contact such as coughing, sneezing, sharing cups, telephones, or toilets, nor will she "give AIDS" to anyone in the course of normal housekeeping. Indeed, she may and should continue to hug her kids. She can continue to cook and clean with normal attention to safety. However, toothbrushes, razors, or other implements that could become contaminated with blood should not be shared and, following incidents that result in bleeding, contaminated surfaces should be cleaned with household bleach freshly diluted with 1 part bleach to 10 parts water. In addition, tampons and sanitary napkins should be carefully disposed of, since menstrual blood does contain the virus.

It is important to stress the hope inherent in this situation and the control the women can exert to avoid moving along the continuum from seropositivity to ARC to AIDS. Women must be made to realize that the exposure to the virus as represented by a positive antibody test does not mean that she will inevitably get the disease of AIDS. There is much she can do to increase her health status. Support groups should be initiated for women who are seropositive. Aside from answering questions and providing emotional support, these groups can focus on the tangible changes a woman can and must make. Checklists, charts, diaries, or journals can be used to give the woman a concrete record of the health maintenance and behavioral changes she needs to make.

Weekly reviews of diaries will help these women stay on track and provide immediate positive feedback, as well as immediate assistance in problem areas. These should start with areas in which the women can experience high rewards and low stress. More difficult issues can then be addressed in a graduated, progressive way on this positive base.

Women will need assistance in discussing their HIV status with partners. Anticipating their discomfort will assist the women in acquiring new skills for coping with this sensitive area. Encouraging role playing and having women share how they have told their partners will give the women opportunities to practice various approaches and find out what feels most comfortable for them. The program should facilitate this communication by offering couple counseling and groups for partners of seropositive clients.

CARE OF THE CHEMICALLY DEPENDENT WOMAN WITH AIDS

The primary care for the chemically dependent woman with AIDS may be the responsibility of medical personnel and the hospital staff. The drug treatment program will have to be integrated with the work of a multidisciplinary team that involves many organizations, including the hospital, child protective services, human resources agencies, and public health departments.

Chemically dependent women will most likely not have the resources to develop the strong support networks seen in the gay communities. For this reason, formal organizations will be essential and primary providers of support for these women. Plans must be made for dependent children prior to the women becoming too debilitated to properly care for them. Drug treatment programs and other agencies may well serve as the lifeline for these women. It is imperative for the well-being of these women, their children, and the rest of society, that the women not slip through the cracks that exist between various service providers.

REFERENCES

Centers for Disease Control. Recommendations for assisting in the prevention of perinatal transmission of HTLV/LAV and AIDS. *MMWR* 34(48): 721-732, 1985.

Centers for Disease Control. Acquired immunodeficiency syndrome (AIDS) among black and Hispanics—United States. *MMWR* 35(42): 655-666, 1986.

Centers for Disease Control. Antibodies to human immunodeficiency virus in female prostitutes. *MMWR* 36(11): 157-161, 1987a.

Centers for Disease Control. Unpublished data, March 9, 1987b.

Centers for Disease Control. *Acquired Immunodeficiency Syndrome (AIDS) Weekly Surveillance Report*. Atlanta: January 4, 1988.

Coates, Thomas J. The impact of AIDS on the sexual behavior of gay men. *Public Health Grand Rounds*. Sacramento: California Department of Health Services, July 11, 1985.

Des Jarlais, D.C.; Chamberland, M.E.; Yancovitz, S.R.; Weinberg, P.; and Friedman, S.R. Heterosexual partners: A large risk group for AIDS. *Lancet* 2(8415):1346-1347, 1984.

Mondanaro, J. Medical services for drug dependent women. In: Beschner, G.M.; Reed, B.G.; and Mondanaro, J., eds. *Treatment Services for Drug Dependent Women*. Vol. I. Rockville, MD: National Institute on Drug Abuse, 1981a. pp. 208-257.

Mondanaro, J. Reproductive health concerns for the treatment of drug dependent women. In: Beschner, G.M.; Reed, B.G.; and Mondanaro, J., eds. *Treatment Services for Drug Dependent Women*. Vol. I. Rockville, MD: National Institute on Drug Abuse, 1981b. pp. 258-292.

Mondanaro, J.; Wedenoja, M.; Densen-Gerber, J.; Elahi, J.; Mason, M.; and Redmond, A. Sexuality and fear of intimacy as barriers to recovery for drug dependent women. In: Reed, B.G.; Beschner, G.M.; and Mondanaro, J., eds. *Treatment Services for Drug Dependent Women*. Vol. II. Rockville, MD: National Institute on Drug Abuse, 1982.

Reed, B.G. Intervention strategies for drug dependent women: An introduction. In: Beschner, G.M.; Reed, B.G.; and Mondanaro, J. *Treatment Services for Drug Dependent Women*. Vol. I. Rockville, MD: National Institute on Drug Abuse, 1981.

Shaw, N.S. California models for women's AIDS education and services. Presented at the American Public Health Association Annual Meeting, Washington, DC, November 20, 1985.

Sutker, P.B. Drug dependent women: An overview of the literature. In: Beschner, G.M.; Reed, B.G.; and Mondanaro, J., eds. *Treatment Services for Drug Dependent Women*. Vol. I. Rockville, MD: National Institute on Drug Abuse, 1981.

Wilsnack, S.C., and Beckman, L.J., eds. *Alcohol Problems in Women*. New York: The Guilford Press, 1984.

AUTHOR

Josette Mondanaro, M.D.
California School of Professional Psychology
5024 Thurber Lane
Santa Cruz, CA 95065

Preventing AIDS: Prospects for Change in White Male Intravenous Drug Users

James L. Sorensen

INTRODUCTION

As 1988 began, it was clear that acquired immunodeficiency syndrome (AIDS) among intravenous drug users (IVDUs) had become a serious problem. Some 49,743 cases of AIDS had been diagnosed: 8,411 among heterosexual IV drug abusers (17 percent) and 3,689 among homosexual/bisexual men (hereafter referred to as gay men) with a history of IV drug abuse (7 percent) (Centers for Disease Control 1987). The National Institute on Drug Abuse estimates that there are approximately 1.1 to 1.3 million IVDUs in the country, of which 200,000 are intermittent users. Of these, the Centers for Disease Control (CDC) estimates that 335,000 are infected with the human immunodeficiency virus (HIV) (Booth 1988).

It was also clear that AIDS among IV drug abusers is a problem not limited to a single ethnic group. Of the 8,411 heterosexual IV drug abusers diagnosed with AIDS, 4,303 (51 percent) are black, 2,394 (28 percent) are Hispanic, and 1,672 (20 percent) are white. In contrast, of the 23,552 AIDS cases among gay men who were not drug abusers, fully 79 percent were white. Bakeman et al. (1987) analyzed the CDC AIDS cases to April 1987 and noted that the number of AIDS cases among heterosexual black and Hispanic male patients using drugs intravenously were 22.6 and 21.4 times higher than the corresponding rate of white male IVDUs. The reasons for the higher rate of cases among black and Hispanic communities are complicated and not fully understood (Bakeman et al. 1986); however, clearly, in the area of AIDS among IV drug abusers, black and Hispanic ethnic groups have been affected disproportionately.

83

By 1991, some 270,000 people in the United States will have AIDS or will have died from the disease; how many others will be infected is uncertain, partly because the virus is spreading into the general population at an unknown rate (Barnes 1986). The proportion of AIDS cases who are IVDUs is expected to remain about the same, with an increase in cases among their sexual partners.

The general public sees drug users as reservoirs of criminality, medical problems, and social ills--a self-destructive lot with few resources. Ginzburg (1984) points out, however, that they are extremely heterogeneous. Preventive interventions are needed and must address the needs of specific racial groups, ethnic backgrounds, sexual preferences, and ages. One theme of this presentation, however, is that the integrity of this constituency must be supported by prevention efforts, not splintered. The hope for prevention lies in unity, both among citizens who use drugs and among those who care about their survival.

This paper focuses on white male heterosexual IVDUs. First, it summarizes the knowledge of HIV infection and AIDS as it applies to this group. Then it discusses community factors that support or hinder the likelihood of performance of preventive behaviors by this group. To document community experiences with related behaviors, the paper comments on experiences with gay men and health promotion campaigns. It also presents anecdotal experiences with HIV-related behaviors, both from the literature and from the author's drug treatment program in San Francisco. Several "second-generation" AIDS prevention models are suggested, and suggestions are made for associated research.

WHAT IS KNOWN ABOUT AIDS FOR DRUG USERS WHO ARE WHITE MALES?

For purposes of this review, population characteristics are separated from behavioral characteristics. The former are defined as factors that describe most study groups, e.g., geographic area, ethnicity and sex, while the latter we define as behaviors that the groups engage in, e.g., needle sharing and drug use.

Population Characteristics

Region. Several studies have found regional variation in rates of infection with HIV. The studies in different regions consistently point to the urban Northeast as an area with an intense

84

concentration of HIV infection among IVDUs. Des Jarlais and
Friedman (1987) point out that the best single predictor of HIV
infection in IVDUs is geographic location. In New York City and
northern New Jersey, the rate of infection among IVDUs has been
estimated to be at least 50 percent (Drucker 1986; Booth 1988).
Studies in 1985 showed that a third of all patients in New Jersey
drug treatment programs tested positive for HIV antibodies (Alcohol,
Drug Abuse and Mental Health Administration 1985). A 1984 study by
Spira et al. (1984) found a seroprevalence rate of 58 percent among
86 IVDUs entering a drug detoxification program. In two studies
with predominantly black and Hispanic IVDUs in New York City,
Brown and Primm (1987) reported seroprevalence of 54 percent among
a group applying for admission to methadone, and 61 percent among a
group in drug treatment for more than a year.

On the West Coast and in most of the rest of the country, HIV is
less widespread among IVDUs. In a 1985 survey, Levy et al. (1986)
found a rate of infection of only 1.7 percent among 345 blood samples from IV drug users attending State-licensed treatment centers in
seven California counties. In a 1984 to 1985 survey in San Francisco,
Chaisson et al. (1987a) found 10 percent of 281 IVDUs recruited from
community-based settings were seropositive. By 1987, the rate of
seroprevalence had risen to 15 percent (Chaisson et al. 1987a). A
study reported by Watters and Cheng (1987) revealed a seroprevalence
rate of 9 percent in 401 IVDUs in San Francisco.

Race. Caucasians have shown lower rates of HIV infection than
ethnic minorities (principally blacks and Hispanics have been studied)
in Manhattan (Cohen et al. 1985; Marmor et al. 1987), the Bronx
(Schoenbaum et al. 1986), Queens (Robert-Guroff et al. 1986), and
San Francisco (Chaisson et al. 1987a). For example, the Chaisson
et al. sample included 51 percent whites and 54 percent men. Racial
differences appeared, as whites had a lower prevalence of seropositivity than blacks and Hispanics, and this finding persisted after
adjusting for needle sharing.

Table 1 presents published studies known to this author that specifically address differences in race and indicators of AIDS risk in their
samples. Ethnic differences appear in three of the six studies, in
each case with whites being less at risk.

Gender and Age. Where sexual differences have been examined,
statistically significant differences have not appeared among IVDUs

(table 1). Nor have studies shown consistent differences in sero-prevalence among different age groups.

TABLE 1. *Summary of published studies: Risk of AIDS among white males relative to other groups*

First Author of Study (Year)	White (Percent)	Men (Percent)	Indicators of AIDS Risks (HIV+, Needle Sharing, Drug Use)
Chaisson (1987a)	51	54	HIV antibodies: less infection in whites. No sex differences in infection. Needle sharing: Fewer whites shared, but those who shared did so with more people.
Dolan (1987)	47	100	Needle sharing: No race differences.
Marmor (1987)	29	74	HIV antibodies: Five racial groups, infected at different rates. Whites' rate = .42; total sample rate = .51. No sex differences.
Robert-Guroff (1986)	34	70	HIV antibodies: Less infection in whites. No sex differences.
Selwyn (1987)	20	53	Knowledge of AIDS: No race or sex differences. Needle sharing: No race or sex differences.
Watters (1987)	51	65	HIV antibodies: No race or sex differences.

Behavioral Characteristics

If every person infected with HIV were to stop engaging in behaviors that spread body fluids, the progression of HIV infection would be stopped completely. Behaviors must be modified to stop AIDS, and behavior changes are crucial. Where IV drug use is concerned, a series of behavioral defenses would stop AIDS. If people want to protect themselves, the best defense is to stop using drugs. A less perfect defense is not to use needles when they take drugs; even less perfect is always to use their own needles and never share; and a last-ditch defense is always to clean the shared needle before using it. A similar set of defenses exist against sexual transmission of AIDS, ranging from abstinence to protecting oneself always with condoms and spermicide. In this section, we examine what is known about these and other behaviors that might put IVDUs at risk.

Injection of Drugs. More frequent injection has been associated with HIV risk consistently in studies in the New York (Marmor et al. 1987) and San Francisco areas (Chaisson et al. 1987a) and also in Dallas (Black et al. 1986, Dolan et al. 1987).

Needle Sharing. Needle sharing seems to be the most important HIV-transmitting behavior among IVDUs; it is implicated in study after study of HIV infection. Needle sharing has been commonplace among IVDUs, even in areas of low seroprevalence. For example, Levy et al. (1986) found that 80 percent of his sample of 345 IVDUs shared. In the Chaisson et al. study (1987b), increased risk of seropositivity was found among addicts who reported regularly sharing needles, especially with two or more people. The study of Brown and Primm (1987) revealed that needle sharing and numbers of people involved with sharing explained more variance in serostatus than race or any other variable.

Because of the importance of needle sharing, several investigators have attempted to understand what factors influence the decision to share. A qualitative study by Des Jarlais et al. (1987b) has explained many of the psychological, social, and cultural reasons that IVDUs share needles. Bakeman et al. (1987) comment that the epidemiology of AIDS may indicate that needle sharing is more widespread among minorities. The evidence for this, however, is mixed. Dolan et al. (1987) surveyed the needle-sharing habits of 224 intakes to a 30-day inpatient drug program in Dallas from 1983 to 1985. Three variables discriminated needle sharers (68 percent of the sample) from other drug abusers: greater severity of drug use, multiple drug use, e.g., opiates and cocaine, and use of shooting galleries. Of the sample, 47 percent were white; race did not predict needle sharing. An earlier study noted that sex roles may make men more likely to use needles on their own (Howard and Borges 1972); needle sharing may be more common among women (Rosenbaum 1981).

Needle Cleaning. Needle hygiene has recently received attention as a "last-ditch" method for an IVDU to prevent HIV infection. Watters and Cheng (1987) found that 87 percent of their sample cleaned needles between sharing partners, but the typical cleaning used tap water (which does not kill HIV) as the cleaning agent.

Obtaining Drug Treatment. In the study of Watters and Cheng (1987) the seroprevalence rate of those out of treatment was about twice that of those who were in treatment for drug use. Sorensen et al. (1988) report large decreases in needle use among seropositive drug abusers once they enter methadone maintenance. However, because of variability in treatment retention, abused drugs, and clientele, it would be naive to expect to see a strong and consistent relationship between drug treatment and risk of contracting or spreading HIV. For example, Hubbard et al. (1988) found that length of time in treatment strongly affects a drug user's AIDS risk.

Prostitution. Two studies in the United States have found that prostitutes are more likely to be infected than other populations (Schoenbaum et al. 1986; Des Jarlais et al. 1987c). On the other hand, in the Chaisson et al. (1987a) study, no association was found between HIV infection and history of prostitution.

Summary

In population characteristics, white male IVDUs living in the Northeast are more likely to be infected than those in other areas of the country. Whites appear to be less likely than blacks or Hispanics to be infected with HIV. Other population characteristics do not consistently predict either HIV infection or risky behaviors. Regarding behavioral characteristics, frequent injection of drugs and needle sharing have been consistently implicated in studies of seroprevalence.

FACTORS THAT AFFECT LIKELIHOOD OF PREVENTION

Several community factors or characteristics may support or hinder the performance of protective and preventive behaviors among white males IVDUs. The factors examined here include cultural differences;

social supports; family background; economic, educational, and psychological resources, and sex role expectations.

Cultural

To the extent that they are better educated, whites more than any other group may benefit from preventive messages in the written media, e.g., newspapers or brochures. Ginzburg et al. (1986) report that in a 1985 New Jersey survey of 577 drug users, more than two-thirds indicated that they had obtained information about AIDS from newspapers, and whites gave positive responses most frequently.

Social Supports

IVDUs have less social support for AIDS risk reduction than do gay males (Friedman et al. 1987). Moss (1986) points out that the drug treatment and AIDS constituencies are almost totally separate, and there has been little evidence of mobilization on the AIDS/IV drug abuse issue anywhere outside the east coast. White males are not thought to differ from other groups in the likelihood that social factors will mitigate risk of HIV infection.

Family

To the extent that white males may be less involved with extended family than are other ethnic groups, they may be more difficult to reach with prevention messages. For males who have a great dependence on their nuclear family, family members may be crucial for AIDS prevention, both as an influence on the drug user and also as targets of preventive information themselves. IVDUs are not typically loners, but have close contacts with their families (Stanton et al. 1982). The spouse and parents of the drug user seem to be the most important significant others that may help in AIDS prevention with white males.

Economic

At the community level, IVDUs generally have few economic re-sources. The community infrastructure that enabled the epidemic among gay men to be treated with substantial volunteer resources is almost totally lacking among IVDUs. The lack of economic resources among IVDUs transcends ethnic and cultural groups and overshadows the economic differences between races or sexes. The lack of economic resources and community infrastructure appears to be the greatest impediment to providing adequate treatment for IVDUs once infection has occurred. Perhaps because whites and males have more money than other IVDUs, they may be less likely to share needles.

Educational/Psychological

If a group is more aware of the threat of AIDS, its members may be less likely to share needles. A study by Selwyn et al. (1987) found that AIDS knowledge predicted less needle sharing among 261 IVDUs in New York. Needle sharers were less likely than nonsharers to have graduated from high school and had lower scores on the AIDS knowledge questionnaire. Hochhauser (1987) evaluated the readability of AIDS educational materials and found the average reading level to be 14th grade, well beyond the comprehension of poorly educated IVDUs. Knowledge may make a difference in AIDS risk. And to the extent that white male IVDUs may be better educated than other groups, they may benefit more from health education efforts.

IV drug use in white males may reflect greater psychological mal-adjustment relative to their cultural norms than is the case of nonwhites. Thus, white males may be less able to make deliberate changes than those whose drug use fits their cultural norm. This appears to be one factor that predicts limited engagement of the white male IVDU in preventive behaviors, the established premise that the higher the social class of an addict, the more likely he or she is suffering from psychopathology (Kaufman 1978).

Sex Roles

A male partner's support may serve as an essential catalyst for safe sexual practices. Men, like women, need social skills training on the use of condoms to overcome any embarrassment they may have in asking a new partner about her sexual practices. As women do, men may believe that condoms remove the spontaneity from sexual activity (Mantel et al., in press). Heterosexual men must learn new sexual repertoires that incorporate condom use. In general, men may be more able than women to determine the use of condoms (Wermuth et al. 1988), because although women can influence condom use, men can control it.

Summary

Some community factors for whites may improve AIDS risk reduction and the benefits from accrued AIDS prevention messages. White males' psychological resources, however, may pose barriers to preventive activities. The special role heterosexual men play in the decisions surrounding sexual encounters is crucial in preventing the spread of AIDS to women. Increasing the likelihood that male IVDUs will use condoms merits serious study.

COMMUNITY EXPERIENCES WITH RELATED BEHAVIORS

Gay Men and AIDS

Experiences with gay men can provide a template for interventions with IVDUs. A study by Stall et al. (1986) showed that use of drugs and alcohol during sex, the number of drugs used during such activity, and the frequency of combining drugs and sex were all positively associated with risky sexual activity for AIDS. In short, they found a strong relationship between drug and alcohol use during sex and noncompliance with safe-sex guidelines. As the group of gay men in San Francisco has changed its norms, the outliers continue to be those with drug and alcohol problems. This experience supports the view of the general public that IVDUs will be unlikely to change their behaviors.

Among gay men, significant changes have occurred in response to the AIDS epidemic. The number of sexual partners and amount of unprotected receptive anal/genital contact have been significantly related to risk of HIV infection (Winkelstein et al. 1987). Significant reductions in these risks have occurred, but risky behaviors have not been eliminated. A survey spanning sexual behavior from 1982 to 1985 among gay men in San Francisco indicated that all forms of sexual activity considered to be high risk for AIDS transmission and reception had decreased substantially (McKusick et al. 1985), but about 25 percent of the sample still reported engaging in at least one sexual act capable of infecting themselves during the month prior to the survey, and 28 percent reported engaging in at least one activity capable of spreading the infection to others. A 1983 survey by McKusick et al. (1985) revealed that gay men attending bathhouses showed little change in number of sex partners, while men in low-risk situations (with few partners or a steady partner) had substantially lowered their frequency of sexual contacts. Knowledge of health guidelines for reducing AIDS risk was quite high among gay men in this study, but this knowledge showed no relation to sexual behavior. In planning AIDS prevention activities among drug abusers, it should be expected that risky behaviors may be lessened, but not eliminated. Programs that increase knowledge of risks will help at first, but once the population is AIDS-aware, more than knowledge will be required to change behaviors.

Further, a study of the determinants of behavioral risk reduction among gay men at risk for AIDS showed that the availability of supportive peer norms was the only variable that was consistently, significantly, and positively related to reducing one's risk of acquiring AIDS (Joseph et al. 1987). Knowledge, perceived threat, and other attitudes toward infection did not make a substantial difference. The implication for IVDUs is that permanent behavior change may not come until IVDUs see that their peer groups' behavioral norms are changing.

Health Promotion Campaigns

Brandt (1988) has pointed to the Federal Government's attempts at syphilis control for guidance in dealing with the AIDS epidemic. He contends that a complicated interplay of forces influences diseases and our social policies for coping with them. There is conflict between the "moral" and the "instrumental" approaches, with the advocates of each approach thinking the other approach promotes infection. Brandt concludes that intensive education programs, widespread provision of condoms, and widespread voluntary confidential testing were useful in fighting the epidemic of syphilis and may provide some insights for contemporary approaches to combat AIDS.

Job (1988) pointed out that in health promotion campaigns the use of fear is often ineffective in achieving the desired behavior change. If a campaign attempts to use fear as part of a punishment procedure, it is unlikely to succeed. To work well, a campaign that uses fear needs to have several elements: (1) fear should occur before a desired behavior is offered; (2) the event upon which the fear is based should appear to be likely; (3) a specific desired behavior should be offered; (4) the level of fear should only be such that the desired behavior offered is sufficient to substantially reduce the fear; and (5) fear offset should occur as a reinforcer for the desired behavior, confirming its effectiveness.

Following these five steps, it can be seen that there are ways in which AIDS prevention campaigns can benefit from this analysis.

(1)   Fear comes first. As AIDS spreads, it seems likely that IVDUs will fear AIDS; however, they do not fear needle sharing, which

is common in the culture. Nor are they likely to believe fear-promoting health educators.

(2)   AIDS is likely. As Moss (1986) has pointed out, HIV presents difficulties because of its slow progression from infection to disease. By the time the first cases appear in a community, the virus will have established a strong hold. Unfortunately, until some cases appear in their neighborhood, it is unlikely that drug abusers will view getting AIDS as a likely event.

(3)   Specific behavior is offered. In San Francisco, an early approach was to give the message "Don't Share," which, although accurate, may have not been specific. It told drug abusers what not to do, but did not offer a specific desired behavior that drug abusers should perform. It was a message of what not to do rather than an action that an IVDU could take. Subsequently, the message has become "Clean your needles with bleach," which is more specific.

(4)   Behavior sufficiently reduces fear. This is unfortunately the opposite side of (3) above. In leading psychoeducational groups of current and former IV drug abusers, the author sees that drug abusers will feel safe only if they have been abstinent and HIV antibody negative for at least 6 months. Giving the message "Clean your needles with bleach" gives them a specific activity to perform, but it does not allay their anxiety (nor should it).

(5)   Fear should stop when the desired behavior is performed. Because the symptoms of AIDS are slow in coming, health promotion campaigns may be presenting the classic-conditioning desensitization paradigm, in which the IVDU is repeatedly presented with a high-risk activity, e.g., sharing needles, without any effective unconditioned stimulus, e.g., no visible signs of HIV infection. Such a scenario allows the addict to discredit the campaign or to deny or rationalize with thoughts such as "I must be immune" or "If it hasn't happened to me yet, it won't."

Summary

Pertinent experiences with the epidemic of AIDS among gay men and with combating the syphilis epidemic imply that educational programs, widespread provision of condoms (and perhaps needles), and wide-spread voluntary confidential antibody testing may contribute to the prevention of AIDS. When contemplating such efforts, however, we should weigh the moral as well as the instrumental viewpoints. AIDS education campaigns that rely on fear seem unlikely to be effective, and may even be counterproductive as they may desensitize their audience to important messages. Planners need guidance in taking advantage of the principles suggested by health education research.

EXPERIENCE WITH HIV-RELATED BEHAVIORS

Behaviors Associated with Transmission

Des Jarlais et al. (1985a) point out that although there are con-siderable barriers to behavior change among addicts, drug users have made some efforts to reduce their risk of acquiring or spreading AIDS. Needle sharing has been an important part of the social con-text of drug use, especially in the initiation into IV drug use, sharing with "running partners" or sexual partners, and sharing in "shooting galleries" (Des Jarlais et al. 1986). The extent of involvement in such needle-sharing behaviors may be directly related to the risk of transmitting or contracting HIV infection.

The author's impression is that AIDS-transmitting sexual activities of drug abusers are more resistant to change than their needle sharing. Like most of the U.S. population, the majority of IVDUs do not use condoms consistently. Discussion in a recent workshop indicated that the resistance of IV drug abusers to using condoms was considerably greater than their resistance to cleaning needles. Those who are sexually active are unlikely to protect their sexual partners from infection. It may be that with male heterosexual IVDUs a better ap-proach is to recommend abstinence. When using opiates, the IVDUs' sexual activity may be restricted anyway, and reinforcing this ten-dency toward sexual inactivity may become a successful way to pre-vent AIDS.

Behaviors Associated with Prevention

Des Jarlais and Friedman (1987) point out that many public officials have concluded that drug users will not change. Yet, as early as 1984, a New York City study showed that drug users in New York knew about AIDS and were more likely to use clean needles (Friedman et al. 1987). Needle sellers reported an increase in demand in 1985 (Des Jarlais et al. 1987c), and were holding bonus sales of drugs to include a free syringe (Des Jarlais and Hopkins 1985). In 1985, Selwyn and colleagues further documented that methadone maintenance patients in New York knew about AIDS and had cut down on their sharing of needles (Selwyn et al. 1987).

In San Francisco, Chaisson et al. (1987a) found that the likelihood that needle sharers usually or always cleaned their needles with bleach grew from 6 percent in 1985 to 47 percent in a 1987 survey. Nonetheless, more than half were not regularly cleaning needles before injecting. Watters (1987) documented an increase in the use of bleach to clean syringes among addicts in San Francisco, from 5 percent in 1986 to 68 percent in 1987. Needle cleaning, though an important component of AIDS prevention, is unlikely to be consistently adopted and is insufficient by itself to stop the further spread of HIV. Nevertheless, it provides evidence that drug users will change their behaviors in response to the threat of AIDS.

The author's experience in a treatment setting has been similar, showing that people only partially change their risk behaviors. Sorensen et al. (1986) found that IVDUs with AIDS or AIDS-related complex (ARC) had problems in the psychological, physical, social support, and confidentiality areas while enrolled in methadone maintenance; however, an evaluation showed drastic reductions in drug usage from before methadone to 3 months into treatment (Sorensen et al. 1988).

SUGGESTED INTERVENTION MODELS

Brandt (1988) points out that no single medical or social intervention can adequately address the problem of the spread of HIV infection. A range of interventions is needed. Table 2 presents possible preventive interventions to change both drug use and sexual behaviors. Community efforts of the early 1980s to prevent youth from advancing to drug use may ultimately have an important preventive effect. For those using drugs, interventions are listed that may reduce needle use. For those using needles, interventions can aim at reducing the likelihood that they will share needles. Finally, for those who share needles, last-stand efforts are needed to encourage needle cleaning. The same approach is presented for preventing the spread of AIDS through sexual behaviors, ranging from interventions that encourage abstinence to programs that will encourage the use of condoms and spermicides—the last defense against AIDS transmission.

TABLE 2. *Suggested intervention models to change HIV-spreading habits*

Drug Use	Sexual Behavior
Prevent Drug Abuse	Encourage Abstinence
Reduce Needle Use	Family and school education
Prevent progression to IV use	Encourage Monogamy*
Make treatment available for IVDUs	Educate sexual partners of IVDUs
Identify high-risks groups for intervention	Use Condoms and Spermicides Properly
Deliver culturally appropriate interventions	Educate IVDUs
Reach out to users not in treatment	Distribute condoms and spermicides
Reduce Needle Sharing	
Educate IVDUs	
Distribute or exchange needles	
Change the needles	
Antibody testing	
Increase Needle Cleaning	
Educate IVDUs	
Distribute bleach and teach	

*It must be noted that monogamy does not offer protection for the regular sexual partner of IV drug abusers.

A number of educational and organizing activities with drug users and the health care network may also help (table 3).

TABLE 3. *Organizational steps to implement interventions*

IVDUs	Health Care Network
Support development of self-help groups	Use drug treatment program staff
Send outreach workers to the streets and galleries	Use AIDS treatment program staff
Send outreach vans	Enlist staff in medical hospitals and clinics
Develop education in treatment programs	Enlist Narcotics Anonymous, Naranon
Develop written materials	
Videos, public service announcements	

Marmor et al. (1984) suggest that some patients with AIDS have been very willing to talk about their disease and their feelings about drug abuse. They have sometimes been able to communicate the hazards of drug abuse and AIDS more effectively than physicians or other medical personnel. We should support the self-organization efforts among IVDUs, if we are to have any hope of changing norms and tapping volunteer resources. Likewise, sending outreach workers in vans to the community may provide education that will not get out through treatment programs.

Drug treatment programs can be centers for AIDS prevention among drug abusers. To the extent that drug treatment reduces the like-lihood that a person will share a needle, treatment is AIDS preven-tion. In addition, it is crucial to develop education in drug treatment programs that provide the most frequent and most trusted contact between social organizations and drug users.

The author's approach has been to develop and evaluate psychoeduca-tional interventions for IVDUs, e.g., 6 hours of group discussion that covers psychological motives and barriers along with education about AIDS. Other preventive activities in San Francisco drug treatment programs have included such activities as supplementing the intake physical examination with information about AIDS, providing bleach and condoms, posting flyers and billboards, distributing brochures, testing for HIV antibodies, showing videotapes, and holding AIDS awareness days.

Although these treatment-based interventions are vital, Watters et al. (1986) point out that policymakers should be sure that treat-ment programs are indeed focusing on AIDS prevention. Specific funds should be allocated for AIDS prevention, rather than allowing funds to trickle down to prevention only after all funding needs of treatment programs have been fully met.

There is also a need to develop media efforts to reach drug users, not just with written materials but with videotapes and public service announcements. In the health care network, staff in drug treatment programs need education about AIDS, and AIDS programs need to prepare to treat drug abusers. In Boston and some other areas, there has been effective liaison with self-help groups for former drug abusers like Narcotics Anonymous or groups for family members, e.g., Naranon. These groups need education to reduce their risks of con-tracting HIV. They may also be used to educate others in their communities, and they may in turn provide the social support that will be so desperately needed.

First-Generation Interventions

It is early in the AIDS epidemic among IVDUs. Creative interventions have been developed, including such activities as AIDS education, antibody testing, clean needle education, some efforts to increase the availability of drug treatment, promotion of condoms, and a limited number of brochures and audiovisual materials. But these alone will not be sufficient.

HIV antibody testing has been suggested as a method not only to track the spread of the epidemic, but to educate IVDUs about AIDS. Carlson and McLellan (1987) point out that such screening is well-accepted by IVDUs in drug treatment programs, and it can be helpful in educating them about the behaviors that spread AIDS. Des Jarlais et al. (1986) found that simply conducting such testing in a treatment program improved the clients' awareness and knowledge of AIDS, even if they did not take the antibody test.

More drug abuse treatment is needed, and more effective treatment is needed, for reducing dependency on drugs. But Newman (1987) points out that treatment needs to be much more available than it has been if IVDUs are to have a realistic opportunity to give up the use of the needle.

Another first-generation educational model is the needle-cleaning education program in San Francisco (Newmeyer et al., in press; Watters et al. 1986). The project team identified a neighborhood where IV drug use was epidemic and identified the needle use patterns that spread HIV. Using that information, an intervention strategy was developed that involved reaching out to IVDUs in the community and teaching them about AIDS and how to clean their injection equipment. Subsequent studies have documented the degree to which that approach "caught on" among IVDUs and spread to those who had not received the outreach contact directly (Chaisson et al. 1987b; Watters 1987).

Second-Generation Interventions

Second-generation interventions aim at specific groups at risk of acquiring or spreading AIDS, or coordinate first-generation approaches more effectively. Although the efficacy of first-generation intervention techniques is unknown, because the AIDS epidemic is moving so quickly, there is no choice but to develop these second-generation efforts before all the data are in.

Des Jarlais and Friedman (1987) emphasize three groups for prevention: (1) those who have not begun IV drug use; (2) those who are willing to enter treatment to eliminate IV drug use; and (3) those who are unwilling to enter treatment and/or for whom present forms of treatment are unlikely to be successful. For those who have not begun drug use, Marmor et al. (1984) pointed out that knowledge of HIV infection rates among IVDUs may be an effective deterrent to beginning the use of a syringe. Similarly, the attitude changes in youth resulting from the parent movement and "just say no" to drugs campaigns may have a long-term effect on the likelihood that future generations will inject drugs. Des Jarlais et al. (1987a) investigated the reasons that drug "sniffers" go on to IV use and have proposed a program to prevent initiation into using needles.

Self-Organization. One model would change the social organization of IV drug use and take advantage of it in interventions (Des Jarlais and Friedman 1985). Self-organization may be the only long-term solution, but it needs much more development before it will be feasible in most communities.

Coordinated Approaches. Moss (1985) has suggested that the combination of antibody testing with availability of drug treatment may do a lot to prevent the spread of AIDS. Specifically, he suggests screening people, finding the HIV positives, and attempting to divert them out of the IV drug use population, or at least out of needle-sharing, before the cases increase rapidly in a community. In short, he recommends finding those people who are seropositive and treating them to prevent spread of the virus, an epidemiologic treatment using the model that worked in syphilis prevention. Such an approach coordinates antibody testing with delivery of effective drug treatment. The approach may be sound epidemiologically, as the provision of treatment to those who test positive would give them something for taking the test, and should be less likely to drive the epidemic underground. The next step would be making treatment for AIDS available to those who test seropositive, e.g., making AZT available to those with an AIDS diagnosis, and perhaps making it available in combination with drug treatment in methadone programs.

AIDS Treatment Interventions. Des Jarlais et al. (1985b) point out that AIDS will create a need for services centered around issues of death and dying. As the number of drug abusers with AIDS increases, there will be a need for more AIDS treatment interventions to deal with depression and grief, to provide more counseling that takes into account neuropsychological deficits, and to offer services for an increasingly ill and homeless population (Batki et al., in press).

SUGGESTIONS FOR ASSOCIATED RESEARCH

The health care problems of the AIDS epidemic strongly suggest the need to understand better how people's health relates to their behavior. Moral exhortation will not be sufficient to slow the epidemic appreciably. Research is needed to identify the most effective approaches to educating groups at risk and changing their risky behavior. Coates et al. (1987) point out that systematic psychosocial research is essential to slow the spread of AIDS.

Ethnographic and Psychological Studies

The need for studies of risky behaviors, why they occur, and how to modify them is well represented in other chapters of this monograph. Such studies are needed of the heterosexual white male drug user as well as with other special community populations. For example, how often do heterosexual white male IVDUs use condoms? Under what conditions do they not use condoms, and why? How can they reliably be persuaded to use condoms consistently? Is it more likely that they will respond to messages that promote abstinence? These kinds of studies are needed for every community group, including white heterosexual male IVDUs.

The following research recommendations apply to all groups of IVDUs, and represent the author's thinking about research that will prevent the spread of HIV among white males and all other IVDUs.

Sample Systematically

Population-based representative studies will never be practical in the underground drug-abusing community. However, improved sampling strategies can be used. Virtually every study of seroprevalence in treatment programs has been based on samples of convenience, rather than on systematically selected groups. More refined methods are needed to establish the degree to which the results of these studies generalize to the treatment population. Similarly, there is a need for studies across geographical areas, using identical methodologies, to establish the degree to which HIV has taken hold in different communities.

Study the Development of Self-Organization

Using what we have learned in the gay community as a template, it appears vital to study self-organization and then to try different models within the IV drug-using community. Without community change, individual change is not likely to be permanent.

Use Existing Educational Models

Preventive educational campaigns should be based upon what has been learned from other health promotion efforts. The health belief model (Rosenstock 1974) has been applied, but it is not clear how effective it is for AIDS prevention. It would be wise to commission a review of the efficacy of such campaigns, both the theory and the specific examples, e.g., smoking and heart disease, and to disseminate this information to health educators to use to prevent the spread of AIDS.

Sow Many Seeds: Develop and Test Interventions

It is vital to develop and test interventions that attempt to prevent the spread of HIV, before infection becomes so widespread that the efforts can focus only on treatment. It would be a mistake to delay intervention studies until the intricacies of risky behavior are fully understood. A range of interventions will need to be developed, then tested rigorously and quickly. Only a few may prove efficacious, but those will be worthy of cross-validation, replication, and immediate dissemination.

Evaluate, Then Disseminate

The field is moving very rapidly, and mistakes are probably being made. For example, there is a widespread assumption that condoms and possibly spermicides can effectively prevent HIV infection, but the evidence for this assumption is not very strong (Feldblum and Fortney 1988). In the drug abuse area, similar mistakes could include recommendations that drug abusers clean their needles with bleach. Seroprevalence studies have not yet shown an association between needle cleaning and avoidance of HIV infection. There is an existing need for more studies on the efficacy of preventive measures and for studies of ways to lengthen the life of those infected. However, it would be a mistake to continue to disseminate purported prevention efforts that have not been shown to be efficacious in objective scientific trials.

Prepare a Dissemination Research Plan

The dissemination/utilization research field should be reviewed to help plan the most effective dissemination strategies. Research literature exists on disseminating interventions (Fairweather and Tornatzky 1977; Glaser et al. 1983) and this should be tapped systematically. Studies will be needed of ways to disseminate the most effective AIDS prevention interventions, and those studies should be started immediately. Dissemination methods should be sharpened now, so they can be used effectively to spread the word about the AIDS prevention techniques that are most effective.

CONCLUSION

A sense of community is necessary to invoke planned social change. In the effort to develop community-based prevention for various groups, innovators should always be cognizant of the overarching goal to prevent the spread of AIDS among IVDUs and from IVDUs to the general population. In this regard, it is important to avoid dividing prevention efforts so that unity gets lost in AIDS prevention campaigns. The tasks of understanding communities, designing AIDS prevention models, creating prevention strategies, evaluating them, and disseminating them to the field provides a challenge for every special community group, including white males. The ultimate challenge will be changing the community norms for all community groups, in concert.

REFERENCES

Alcohol, Drug Abuse and Mental Health Administration. AIDS studied among drug users. *ADAMHA News,* November 1985. pp. 1-2.

Bakeman, R.; Lumb, J.R.; Jackson, R.E.; and Smith, D.W. AIDS risk group profiles in whites and members of minority groups. *N Engl J Med* 315:3, 1986.

Bakeman, R.; McCray, E; Lumb, J.R.; Jackson, R.E.; and Whitley, P.N. The incidence of AIDS among blacks and Hispanics. *J Natl Med Assoc* 79:921-928, 1987.

Barnes, D.M. Grim projections for AIDS epidemic. *Science* 232:1589-1590, 1986.

Batki, S.L.; Sorensen, J.L.; Faltz, B.; and Madover, S. AIDS among drug abusers: Psychiatric aspects of treatment. *Hosp Community Psychiatry,* in press.

Black, J.L.; Dolan, M.P.; DeFord, H.A.; Rubenstein, J.A.; Penk, W.E.; Robinowitz, R.; and Skinner, J.R. Patterns of needle sharing among intravenous drug abusers. Presented at the meeting of the American Psychological Association, Washington, DC, August 1986.

Booth, W. CDC paints a picture of HIV infection in US. *Science* 239:253, 1988.

Brandt, A.M. The syphilis epidemic and its relation to AIDS. *Science* 239:375-380, 1988.

Brown, L.S., and Primm, B.J. AIDS infection among blacks and Hispanics: The role of intravenous drug user in the racial distribution of AIDS. Presented at the meeting of the American Public Health Association, October 1987.

Carlson, G.A., and McLellan, T.A. The voluntary acceptance of HIV-antibody screening by intravenous drug users. *Public Health Rep* 102(4):391-394, 1987.

Centers for Disease Control. *AIDS Weekly Surveillance Report–United States.* December 28, 1987.

Chaisson, R.E.; Moss, A.R.; Onishi, R.; Osmond, D.; and Carlson, J.R. Human immunodeficiency virus infection in heterosexual intravenous drug users in San Francisco. *Am J Public Health* 77(2):169-172, 1987a.

Chaisson, R.E.; Osmond, D.; Moss, A.R.; Feldman, H.W.; and Biernacki, P. HIV, bleach, and needle sharing. *Lancet* 8547(1):1430, 1987b.

Coates, T.J.; Stall, R.; Mandel, J.S.; Boccellari, A.; Sorensen, J.L.; Morales, E.F.; Morin, S.F.; Wiley, J.A.; and McKusick, L. AIDS: A psychosocial research agenda. *Annals of Behavioral Medicine* 9(2):21-28, 1987.

Cohen, H.; Marmor, M.; Des Jarlais, D.C.; Spira, T.; Friedman, S.R.; and Yancovitz, S. Risk factors for HTLV-III/LAV seropositivity among intravenous drug users. Presented at the International Conference on AIDS, Atlanta, April 1985.

Des Jarlais, D.C., and Friedman, S.R. Prevention policy questions for AIDS among intravenous drug users. Presented at the meeting of the American Public Health Association, Washington, DC, November 1985.

Des Jarlais, D.C.; Friedman, S.R.; and Hopkins, W. Risk reduction for the acquired immunodeficiency syndrome among intravenous drug users. *Ann Intern Med* 103:755-759, 1985a.

Des Jarlais, D.C., and Hopkins, W. Free needles for intravenous drug users at risk for AIDS: Current developments in New York City. *N Engl J Med* 323:1476, 1985.

103

Des Jarlais, D.C.; Jainchill, N.; and Friedman, S.R. AIDS among IV drug users: Epidemiology, natural history, and therapeutic community experiences. Presented at the World Conference of Therapeutic Communities, San Francisco, CA, September 1985b.

Des Jarlais, D.; Friedman, S.; Marmor, M.; and Cohen, H. AIDS and behavior change among intravenous drug users. Presented at the meeting of the American Psychological Association, Washington, DC, August 1986.

Des Jarlais, D.C., and Friedman, S.R. HIV infection among intravenous drug users: Epidemiology and risk reduction. *AIDS Int J* 1(2):67-76, 1987.

Des Jarlais, D.C.; Friedman, S.R.; Casriel, C.; and Kott, A. AIDS and preventing initiation into intravenous (IV) drug use. *Psychol Health* 1(2):179-194, 1987a.

Des Jarlais, D.C.; Friedman, S.R.; and Strug, D. AIDS and needle sharing within the IV-drug use subculture. In: Feldman, D.A., and Johnson, T.M., eds. *The Social Dimensions of AIDS.* New York: Praeger, 1987b. pp. 111-125.

Des Jarlais, D.C.; Wish, E.; Friedman, S.R.; Stoneburner, R.; Yancovitz, S.; Mildvan, D.; El-Sadr, W.; Brady, E.; and Cuadrado, M. Intravenous drug use and heterosexual transmission of human immunodeficiency virus: Current trends in New York City. *NY State J Med* 87:283-285, 1987c.

Dolan, M.P.; Black, J.L.; DeFord, H.A.; Skinner, J.R.; and Robinowitz, R. Characteristics of drug abusers that discriminate needle-sharers. *Public Health Rep* 102(4):395-397, 1987.

Drucker, E. AIDS and addiction in New York City. *Am J Drug Alcohol Abuse* 12:165-181, 1986.

Fairweather, G.W., and Tornatzky, L.G. *Experimental Methods for Social Policy Research.* New York: Pergamon, 1977. 420 pp.

Feldblum, P.J., and Fortney, J.A. Condoms, spermicides, and the transmission of human immunodeficiency virus: A review of the literature. *Am J Public Health* 78(1):52-54, 1988.

Friedman, S.R.; Des Jarlais, D.C.; Sotheran, J.L.; Garber, J.; Cohen, H.; and Smith, D. AIDS and self-organization among intravenous drug users. *Int J Addict* 22:201-220, 1987.

Ginzburg, H.M. Intravenous drug users and the acquired immune deficiency syndrome. *Public Health Rep* 99(2):206-212, 1984.

Ginzburg, H.M.; French, J.; Jackson, J.; Hartsock, P.I.; MacDonald, M.G.; and Weiss, S.H. Health education and knowledge assessment of HTLV-III diseases among intravenous drug users. *Health Educ Q* 13(4):373-382, 1986.

Glaser, E.M.; Abelson, H.H.; and Garrison, K.N. *Putting Knowledge to Use: Facilitating the Diffusion of Knowledge and the Implementation of Planned Change.* San Francisco: Jossey-Bass, 1983. 636 pp.

Hochhauser, M. Readability of AIDS educational materials. Presented at the meeting of the American Psychological Association, New York, August 1987.

Howard, J., and Borges, P. Needle-sharing in the Haight: Some social and psychological functions. In: Smith, D.B., and Gay, G., eds. *It's So Good, Don't Even Try it Once.* Englewood Cliffs, NJ: Prentice-Hall, 1972. pp. 125-136.

Hubbard, R.L.; Marsden, M.E.; Cavanaugh, E.; Rachal, J.V.; and Ginzburg, H.M. Role of drug-abuse treatment in limiting the spread of AIDS. *Rev Infect Dis* 10(2):377-384, 1988.

Job, R.F.S. Effective and ineffective use of fear in health promotion campaigns. *Am J Public Health* 78(2):163-167, 1988.

Joseph, J.G.; Montgomery, S.B.; Emmons, C.A.; Kessler, R.C.; Ostrow, D.C.; Wortman, C.B.; O'Brien, K.; Eller, M.; and Eshleman, S. Magnitude and determinants of behavioral risk reduction: Longitudinal analysis of a cohort at risk for AIDS. *Psychol Health* 1:73-96, 1987.

Kaufman, E. The relationship of social class and ethnicity to drug abuse. In: Smith, D.E.; Anderson, S.M.; Boyton, M.; Gottlieb, N.; Harvey, W.; and Chung, T., eds. *A Multicultural View of Drug Abuse: Proceedings of the National Drug Abuse Conference, 1977.* Cambridge, MA: Schenkman, 1978. pp. 158-164.

Levy, N.; Carlson, J.R.; Hinrichs, S.; Lerche, N.; Schenker, M.; and Gardner, M.B. The prevalence of HTLV-III/LAV antibodies among intravenous drug users attending treatment programs in California: A preliminary report. *New Engl J Med* 314(7):446, 1986.

Mantel, J.E.; Schinke, S.P.; and Akabas, S.H. Women and AIDS prevention. *J Primary Prev*, in press.

Marmor, M.; Des Jarlais, D.C.; Cohen, H.; et al. Risk factors for infection with human immunodeficiency virus among intravenous drug abusers in New York City. *AIDS Int J* 1(1):39-44, 1987.

Marmor, M.; Des Jarlais, D.C.; Friedman, S.R.; Lyden, M.; and El-Sadr, W. The epidemic of acquired immunodeficiency syndrome (AIDS) and suggestions for its control in drug abusers. *J Subst Abuse Treat* 1:237-247, 1984.

McKusick, L. and Coates, T.J. Behaviors associated with receiving and transmitting the HTLV-III virus among gay men in San Francisco: The AIDS behavioral research project. University of California, San Francisco, 1986. Unpublished manuscript.

McKusick, L.; Horstman, W.; and Coates, T.J. AIDS and sexual behavior reported by gay men in San Francisco. *Am J Pub Health* 75:493-496, 1985.

Moss, A.M. New risk groups in AIDS. Paper presented at the meeting of the American College of Epidemiology, Santa Monica, CA, September 1985.

Moss, A.M. AIDS in IV drug users. Paper presented at the New Jersey State Health Department meeting on AIDS in the IV drug using community, April 1986.

Newman, R.G. Methadone treatment: Defining and evaluating success. *N Engl J Med* 317(7):447-450, 1987.

Newmeyer, J.A.; Feldman, H.W.; Biernacki, P.; and Watters, J.K. Preventing AIDS contagion among intravenous drug users. *Med Anthropol*, in press.

Robert-Guroff, M.; Weiss, S.H.; Giron, J.A.; Jennings, A.M.; Ginzburg, H.M.; Margolis, I.B.; Blattner, W.A.; and Gallo, R.C. Prevalence of antibodies to HTLV-I, -II, and -III in intravenous drug users from an AIDS endemic region. *JAMA* 255:21-25, 1986.

Rosenbaum, M. Sex roles among deviants: The woman addict. *Int J Addict* 16(5):859-877, 1981.

Rosenstock, I.M. The health belief model and preventive health behavior. *Health Education Monographs* 2(4):355-385, 1974.

Schoenbaum, E.E.; Selwyn, P.A.; Klein, R.S.; Rogers, M.F.; Freeman, K.; and Friedland, G.H. Prevalence of and risk factors associated with HTLV-III/LAV antibodies among intravenous drug abusers in methadone programs in New York City. Presented at the International Conference on AIDS, Paris, June 1986.

Selwyn, P.A.; Feiner, C.; Cox, C.P.; Lipschutz, C.; and Cohen, R.L. Knowledge about AIDS and high-risk behaviors among intravenous drug users in New York City. *AIDS Int J* 1:247-254, 1987.

Sorensen, J.L.; Batki, S.L.; Coates, C.; and Gibson, D.R. Methadone maintenance as AIDS prevention: Efficacy three months into treatment. Paper presented at the meeting of the American Public Health Association, Boston, MA, November 1988.

Sorensen, J.L.; Batki, S.L.; Faltz, B.; and Madover, S. Treatment of AIDS in substance abuse programs. Poster presented at the meeting of the American Psychological Association, Washington, DC, August 1986.

Spira, T.J.; Des Jarlais, D.C.; Marmor, M.; Yancovitz, S.; Friedman, S.; Garber, J.; Cohen, H.; Cabradillo, C.; and Kalyanaraman, V.C. Prevalence of antibody to lymphadenopathy-associated virus among drug detoxification patients in New York. *N Engl J Med* 311(7): 467-468, 1984.

Stall, R.; McKusick, L.; Wiley, J.; Coates, T.J.; and Ostrow, D.G. Alcohol and drug use during sexual activity and compliance with safe sex guidelines for AIDS: The AIDS behavioral research project. *Health Educ Q* 12:359-371, 1986.

Stanton, M.D.; Todd, T.C., and associates. *The Family Therapy of Drug Abuse and Addiction.* New York: Guilford, 1982.

Watters, J.K. Preventing human immunodeficiency virus contagion among intravenous drug users: The impact of street-based education on risk behavior. Presented at the Third International Conference on AIDS, Washington, DC, June 1987.

Watters, J.K., and Cheng, Y.T. HIV-1 infection and risk among intravenous drug users in San Francisco: Preliminary results and implications. *Contemporary Drug Problems* 14:411-423, 1987.

Watters, J.K.; Newmeyer, J.A.; Feldman, H.W.; and Biernacki, P. Street-based AIDS prevention for intravenous drug users in San Francisco: Prospects, options, and obstacles. In: *Community Epidemiology Work Group Proceedings June 1986.* Vol. II. National Institute on Drug Abuse administrative report, 1986. pp. 37-43.

Wermuth, L.; Ham, J.; and Gibson, D.R. AIDS prevention outreach to female partners of IV drug users. Presented at the meeting of the American Public Health Association, Boston, MA, November 1988.

Winkelstein, W.; Lyman, D.M.; Padian, N.; et al. Sexual practices and risk of infection by the human immunodeficiency virus. *JAMA* 257:321-325, 1987.

ACKNOWLEDGMENTS

This project was supported by U.S. Public Health Service grant DA 04340 from the National Institute on Drug Abuse and grant MH 42459 from the National Institute of Mental Health and National Institute on Drug Abuse to the University of California, San Francisco.

AUTHOR

James L. Sorensen, Ph.D.
Adjunct Professor and
    Chief, Substance Abuse Services
Department of Psychiatry
University of California, San Francisco
Substance Abuse Services - Ward 92
UCSF at San Francisco General Hospital
1001 Potrero Avenue
San Francisco, CA 94110

Sexual Minority Needle Users

A. Billy S. Jones

INTRODUCTION

Initially, the focus of this paper was to be on "gay IV drug users."
However, the term "gay" is a term more often used to refer to men
who have exclusive relationships with men, thereby excluding bisexual
men and women, lesbians, and transpersons (transsexuals, transvestites, transgenders, crossdressers, and male or female impersonators).
Whereas "gay" is used by some to refer to men and women who pre-
fer same-gender relationships, the term "sexual minority" is more
inclusive of diverse lifestyles and orientations that deviate from
heterosexuality.

The term "intravenous drug user" (IVDU) does not take into consideration the practice of skin popping and intramuscular injecting, which
are also high-risk activities for human immunodeficiency virus (HIV)
infection. Since addicts are often looking for ways to exclude themselves from HIV at-risk behaviors and ways to continue the use of
narcotics, it is important to use terms that are as inclusive of addict
subcultures as possible. Thus, "needle drug user" (NDU) may be a
more inclusive and appropriate term than "intravenous drug user."

WHO ARE SEXUAL MINORITIES—GAYS?

While sexual minorities (gays) are by no means a homogeneous group,
they are a part of every ethnic, racial, socioeconomic, religious, and
community group. Like racial minority communities, sexual minority
communities are more prevalent and visible in large metropolitan
cities. Such cities contain diverse lifestyles, offer pluralistic social
settings, and assure civil and human rights protection to their
residents (Holloran 1970). New York, San Francisco, Los Angeles,

Houston, the District of Columbia, Newark, Miami, and Chicago are examples of cities that have the highest incidence of HIV infection among needle users as well as a large population of sexual minorities. Because of the often closed and secretive nature of subculture communities, effective outreach is difficult.

Lesbians

In many cities, community health outreach workers have identified 1 to 3 percent of their contacts as self-identified lesbians or bisexual women who are engaged in prostitution and may be substance abusers sharing needles. Drug treatment programs see a small percentage of lesbian/bisexual women concerned about HIV infection because they are not far removed from a male relationship and have a history of sharing needles. Alternative Test Sites note that some women receiving HIV-positive test results are self-identified lesbians or bisexuals who are often recovering or practicing NDUs (Jones and Izzo 1988).

Transpersons

While many transpersons do not identify themselves as gay or bisexual (in fact, research indicates that the majority of transvestites and transsexuals are heterosexuals), this is a population that is often overlooked or scorned by gay and nongay communities (Weinberg and Williams 1974). In large metropolitan cities, community health outreach workers have found that it is not unusual to locate visible subcultures of transpersons who are involved in prostitution and have a history of needle drug use and needle sharing (Jones and Izzo 1988). There are also significant numbers of transpersons who are enmeshed in mainstream subcultures and not readily identified. In terms of social stigma and potential legal harassment, transpersons may more closely identify with lesbian/gay communities (Raymond 1979).

Married

Lesbians, gays, bisexuals, and transpersons constitute an often overlooked sexual minority who embrace heterosexual marriage and may also be parents (Weinberg and Williams 1974). Although we have no means of knowing how large this subculture may be or to what extent this subculture may be involved in at-risk HIV-infection activities, we do know, through the presence of lesbian/gay married support groups, and bisexual support groups, that their numbers are significant. While some partners are aware of their spouse's bisexuality, many are not (Wolff 1977). To what extent substance abuse and, more specifically, needle sharing exist in these subcultures is not known; however, acquired immunodeficiency syndrome (AIDS) education messages must be aimed at these persons who may more closely identify with mainstream communities than with lesbian/gay communities.

Situational Bisexuality

While many persons may admit to an occasional relationship or sexual encounter with a person of the same gender, they may very readily reject the clinical and social labels that define them as sexual minorities (Blackwood 1986), in much the same manner that persons who occasionally are involved in needle drug use may reject labels of "addict" or "IVDU."

Men and Women Incarcerated or Otherwise Institutionalized

Incarcerated or institutionalized men and women may express their sexuality through same-gender relationships while in these settings but return to heterosexual relationships upon release. The sharing of needles for drugs, tattoos, and ear piercing may be a part of these bonding relationships. Although prohibited, drugs are smuggled into institutionalized settings, and needle sharing becomes a part of the bonding that bring gays and nongays together (Wooden and Parker 1982). It is not unusual to find homemade needles that are shared by dozens of persons who have no means of acquiring new sets of works and little knowledge of how to sterilize works in settings that do not offer bleach, alcohol, or boiling water. And while institutionalized gays and nongays may know that, barring abstinence, latex condoms and waterbased lubricants are the best tools to protect oneself against HIV infection, these tools are often prohibited in such settings as prisons, detention centers, jails, mental institutions, boarding schools, and residential drug programs (National Academy of Sciences 1986).

Men and Women in Commercialized Sex Industries (Prostitutes and Hustlers)

Participants in commercial sex may be involved in same-gender relationships and encounters as well as heterosexual relationships and encounters. The labels "lesbian," "gay," or "bisexual" may never be embraced, but many of the men and women involved in prostitution state that some of their most meaningful and caring relationships have come from persons of the same gender; yet they adamantly state that they are heterosexuals. The observation of outreach workers is that most persons in the commercialized sex industries are very aware and conscientious about reducing their risk for HIV infection via sexual activities but are not as aware or conscientious about reducing their risk for HIV infection via drug needle sharing. While the overwhelming majority of prostitutes and hustlers identify themselves as heterosexuals, some do identify themselves as lesbian, gay, or bisexual, but they may engage in heterosexual relationships and may be sharing needles with heterosexual partners (Jones and Izzo 1988).

Sexual Minority Youth

Whereas a great amount of AIDS education and outreach is directed toward youth, very seldom are sexual minority youth acknowledged. Yet, we know that many youth get in touch with their sexuality and experiment with sex and drugs at very early ages (Charna 1986). Thus, we must focus on sexuality and substance abuse issues in ways that will not isolate or stigmatize gay and lesbian youth. It is not unusual to learn that persons involved in prostitution and IV drug use/needle drug use began these activities when they were adolescents. Because of the myth that gays are child molesters (in fact, 90 percent of all child molestation is committed by heterosexual males) (Tsang 1981), many sexual minority organizations will not provide services (such as HIV antibody testing or treatment for venereal disease) to persons under the age of 21 or 18.

Partners of Sexual Minority NDUs

Often, lesbians, gays, and transpersons are assumed to be "single." Or, because of the stigma attached to being a sexual minority, partners of sexual minorities are often excluded from efforts to educate partners of IVDUs/NDUs. To the same extent that efforts must be made to educate heterosexual partners of IVDUs/NDUs about risk factors for HIV infection, programs must be developed for partners of sexual minorities. Many sexual minorities who have a history of needle drug use have been in long-term relationships and should be acknowledged as "couples" (and in cases of parenting status, as "families") to the same extent that we acknowledge heterosexual couples and families (Finnegan and McNally 1987).

Since sexual minorities and NDUs are often not visible but are indeed a part of every subculture, all AIDS education efforts must include messages that focus on the behavior of sexual minorities and NDUs. Gay communities must not only focus on mainstream gays who are politically astute and comfortable with their sexuality, but must net-work with communities, agencies, and institutions to reach sexual minorities who identify more closely with other subcultures. Risk-reduction messages must have as much focus on safer needle and drug paraphernalia use as on safer sex practices. To the same extent that we assume that everyone "potentially" may have engaged in some at-risk behavior for HIV infection, we must assume that every sub-culture "potentially" includes sexual minorities as well as current or recovering NDUs (Hawley, unpublished manuscript).

INCIDENCE OF SUBSTANCE ABUSE IN THE LESBIAN/GAY COMMUNITY

While the Weekly Surveillance Report of the Centers for Disease Control (CDC) shows that about 7 percent of persons diagnosed with AIDS had dual transmission risk of homosexuality and needle drug use (Centers for Disease Control 1988), a much higher incidence of other forms of substance abuse may be contributing to the progression of HIV infection. Thus, AIDS education efforts must acknowledge and address nonneedle-using substance abuse as a possible cofactor within sexual minority communities.

A 1975 survey by the Los Angeles Gay Community Services Center revealed that persons patronizing lesbian and gay bars spend an average of 80 percent of their social activities time in bars, discos, and establishments where alcohol is served (Fifield 1975). Whereas an updated survey in the eighties is likely to reveal that persons patronizing lesbian and gay bars are spending less than 80 percent of their time in such social settings, such a survey may also reveal that the trafficking and use of other drugs (including cocaine, heroin, dilaudid, methamphetamine, quaaludes, valium, and marijuana) is not uncommon. In addition, it is not uncommon to observe patrons in lesbian and gay social settings sharing drug paraphernalia.

Considering the social role of bars, taverns, and clubs in lesbian and gay communities, it is not surprising that researchers (Morales and Graves 1988) have found the incidence of alcohol dependence to be higher (25 to 35 percent) among sexual minorities than in the general population (10 percent). Beyond hypothesizing, very little research has focused on the drug patterns of sexual minorities. The lack of reliable information makes decisions about health and drug treatment services for sexual minority communities difficult. Often, conclusions have been made on the basis of assumptions and myths about lesbians, gays, and transpersons that have little or no basis in fact (Weathers 1981). The absence of information about drug use among gay men can impede critical public health intervention efforts. Because of the lack of baseline data, it is difficult to allocate funds or develop appropriate drug treatment services for sexual minorities.

Based on the high incidence of alcoholism in the lesbian and gay communities and the social settings of sexual minorities that embrace drugs and alcohol, some researchers hypothesize that drug use may actually be higher among lesbians and gays than has been documented among their heterosexual counterparts (Caputo 1985). Drug treatment programs that target sexual minorities (Weathers 1981; Morales 1988; Ziebold 1980) have found a pattern of polydrug use, with alcohol being the significant second substance of choice. The choice of drugs among sexual minorities seems to be influenced by availability and locale, by socioeconomic group, and by racial/ethnic group. While the amphetamines and cocaine seem to be the most popular drugs in lesbian and gay communities, a much higher use of heroin is noted among sexual minorities who are street-oriented racial minorities. It is the observation of outreach workers that sexual-minority heroin addicts are more closely identified with the main-stream drug subculture than with the lesbian/gay community.

AIDS AWARENESS AMONG SEXUAL MINORITY IVDUs/NDUs

Because of the extensive focus on the gay community regarding AIDS and the response of the gay community to the AIDS crisis, most gay men are aware that certain sexual behaviors may put them at risk for HIV infection. However, most of the AIDS education messages aimed at the gay community focus on sexual transmission risk factors and not needle drug use transmission factors. Very little AIDS education is directed toward IVDUs/NDUs. Until 1986, CDC's Weekly Surveil-lance Reports did not have a category for "homosexual male and IV drug abuser"; thus, many persons did not recognize that they might be engaging in multiple risk behaviors for HIV infection.

Many sexual minorities do not have access to services of the gay community, especially if they do not live in a major metropolitan area (Ziebold 1980). Others (especially racial minorities) may not identify strongly with the gay community and may seldom read gay publica-tions or attend gay political and social functions. While the gay community as a whole has done an excellent job of reaching, educating, and changing the attitudes and behaviors of those sexual minorities who have close ties to the gay community, there remain class, racial, gender, and social barriers that have rendered the gay community's outreach and education efforts ineffective for some persons (Jones and Izzo 1988; Hawley, unpublished manuscript).

Many lesbians believe they are not at risk for HIV infection. Yet outreach workers do identify women who are IVDUs/NDUs, engaged in prostitution, or not very far removed from male relationships (Jones and Izzo 1988). Sexual minorities in heterosexual marriages and lesbian/gay youth have not been specifically targeted by most AIDS prevention programs. The gay community still seems baffled about how to reach those lesbians and gays who are also racial minorities with strong emotional ties to black, Latina/Hispanic, Asian, or Native-American communities.

Because there are social stigmas attached to being identified as a sexual minority as well as to being identified as an IVDU/NDU, many persons who may fit more than one at-risk category often do not acknowledge one or the other until they are thoroughly familiar with support services. Consider the social stigma regarding homosexuality as opposed to drug use. Consider the strong belief in many communities that AIDS is a "gay disease" (initially, AIDS was referred to as GRID--gay-related immune deficiency). In many subcultures, there is less stigma attached to having a history of IV drug use/needle drug use than a lifestyle and orientation of homosexuality. Thus, many persons initially deny that they are gay or have ever engaged in a same-gender relationship, but admit to IV drug use (some persons with AIDS even "invent" histories of IV drug use, relationship with a prostitute, or a blood transfusion years ago).

In the era of AIDS, many persons who are identified as gay may find themselves banned from "oil joints" (drug shooting galleries or get-off joints) and distanced from heterosexual IVDUs/NDUs except to "cop" or purchase drugs. Many gays are refused admission to residential drug treatment programs because of homophobia and/or AIDS-phobia in addition to the false assumption that all gays have AIDS or that HIV can be transmitted by casual contact. Persons identifying themselves as gay or bisexual risk being distanced from their families and losing support services. Thus, many IVDUs/NDUs seeking services at social service agencies often do not initially identify themselves as a sexual minority. Many gay and bisexual clients seeking services at clinics and social service agencies do not initially profess to a history of IV drug use or other substance abuse. Service providers must take these attitudes into account and include messages about sexuality and substance abuse in all messages to all clients.

ATTITUDES AND AWARENESS ABOUT RISK-REDUCTION MESSAGES

Many substance abuse counselors and administrators maintain judgmental and restrictive attitudes toward sexual minorities. Homosexuality is still viewed by many drug treatment professionals as a pathology even though professional associations such as the American Psychological Association, the American Psychiatric Association, and the National Association of Social Workers have repeatedly stated that homosexuality "per se" is not a pathology. Such negative attitudes, even when disguise is attempted, seriously hinder the recovery from drug addiction of sexual minorities.

Some residential drug treatment programs state that the client's sexual orientation is a major problem and make efforts to change the person's orientation rather than addressing negative behavior that may hinder recovery. Thus, the sexual minority's chances for recovery may range from poor to nonexistent.

While there appears to be a national push for therapeutic drug programs to test clients for HIV antibodies or HIV infection, many of the residential programs wish to test clients for the negative purpose of excluding those who are seropositive.

The gay community has been at the forefront of AIDS education efforts to reduce HIV infection not only among gay men, but also within the mainstream population. However, much of the emphasis of AIDS education messages from gay groups is on sexual issues with very little emphasis on the very real possibility of HIV infection via shared drug paraphernalia. Risk-reduction messages regarding drug paraphernalia have only recently begun to surface within the subcultures of transpersons, youth, and prostitutes.

A survey (Jones 1988) conducted in 1987 by health educators at the Whitman-Walker Clinic's Sunnye Sherman AIDS Education Project revealed that:

- Of 250 persons applying to be volunteers (mostly middle-class white gay men), 78 percent did not know that sharing cookers, dirty water, and filters could be a transmission factor for HIV infection; and

115

- 78 percent knew about the risks of sharing needles and syringes.

A survey (Jones 1988) of 375 men and women incarcerated in the metropolitan Washington, DC, area revealed that prior to education seminars:

- 89 percent did not know about the danger of sharing cookers, water, and filters, but did know that sharing needles was risky;

- 11 percent said that they did not know that HIV infection was possible from needles and syringes, but did know about sexual risks;

- 24 percent insisted that only gay men were at risk for HIV infection and only 2 percent thought that lesbians may be involved in at-risk behavior for HIV infection;

- 17 percent of the male inmates admitted to having "gotten off" with a man (usually stating that they were on the receiving end of oral sex) over the last 10 years, while only 6 percent of the male inmates professed to be gay or bisexual;

- 22 percent of the women professed to having "fooled around" with another woman, and 9 percent professed to bisexuality. Yet, none of the women in this survey defined themselves as a lesbian;

- 91 percent of the inmates had a history of drug use and/or prostitution. However, the survey did not distinguish needle drug use from nonneedle use;

- Only 3 percent of the inmates knew about cleaning works with bleach, while all of those inmates who professed to needle drug use stated that they made some effort to clean their works (flushing with water or alcohol);

- 51 percent of the inmates stated that they never shot up after another person but would pass their works on to another NDU, and only 8 percent stated that they would not pass their works to another shooting partner;

- 92 percent of the inmates felt that, if they knew the symptoms of AIDS, they could look at a person and tell if that person had AIDS, while 97 percent believed that having AIDS and being HIV infected meant the same thing: death; and

- 89 percent of the inmates surveyed revealed that if they discovered that they had AIDS, AIDS-related complex (ARC), or were HIV infected they would attempt suicide via overdose of drugs.

CONCLUSION

The IV-drug-using/needle-drug-using communities are not going to be easy to reach. Like the nongay IVDU/NDU, sexual minority IVDUs/ NDUs are neither monolithic nor homogeneous. HIV risk-reduction programs (outreach, education, counseling and seminar services, treatment) for sexual minority NDUs must recognize that needs may differ along boundaries of race, socioeconomic class, marital/ relationship status, urban vs. rural settings, and degree of openness about sexual orientation and lifestyle (overt vs. covert). To the same extent that service providers must make efforts to work through racism and sexism, efforts must be made to acknowledge and work through homophobia.

Since IVDUs/NDUs communicate mainly by word of mouth, one-on-one efforts to reach and teach sexual minority addicts must be encouraged. There are needs for more subcultural outreach and educational efforts; within given communities subcultures within subcultures must be acknowledged. Thus, what works for the transperson community may not work for the male hustler's community or the married bisexual living in the suburbs.

Drug paraphernalia laws that prohibit purchase of syringes and needles and laws that incarcerate persons for being in possession of drug paraphernalia should be examined. While risk-reduction messages are saying one thing, legislation is imposing another. Persons are addicts because of the substances they put into their bodies, but HIV infection is a reality if addicts share needles, syringes, cotton, and cookers.

To the same extent that partners of nongay IVDUs being at risk for HIV infection are acknowledged, "significant others" of lesbians, gays, and transpersons should also be acknowledged.

There is a need for residential drug treatment programs to have treatment modalities specifically for sexual minorities. Currently, there are no residential drug treatment programs for sexual minorities and only three such programs for recovering alcoholics (Pride Institute in Minnesota, Right Step in Oregon, and Mountain Wood in

Virginia). Until residential drug treatment programs are in place that respect the emotional and cultural needs of sexual minorities who are recovering addicts, existing drug treatment programs must make efforts to confront and address homophobia and gender bias among staff as well as clients.

REFERENCES

Blackwood, E. *The Many Faces of Homosexuality: Anthropological Approaches to Homosexual Behavior.* New York: Harrington Park Press, 1986.

Caputo, L. Dual diagnosis: AIDS and addiction. *Social Work* Vol. 30, No. 4. NASW, July-August, 1985. pp. 361-364.

Centers for Disease Control. *AIDS Weekly Surveillance Report.* Atlanta: March 21, 1988.

Charna, K. *Counseling Our Own: The Lesbian/Gay Subculture Meets The Mental Health System.* Renton, WA: Publication Services, 1986.

Fifield, L. *On My Way To Nowhere: An Analysis of Gay Alcohol Abuse and an Evaluation of Alcoholism Rehabilitation Services of the Los Angeles Gay Community.* Los Angeles: County of Los Angeles, 1975.

Finnegan, D.G., and McNally, E.B. *Dual Identities: Counseling Chemically Dependent Gay Men and Lesbians.* Center City, MN: Hazelden Educational Materials, 1987.

Hawley, P. Epidemiology of AIDS in gay men and IV drug users. February, 1988, unpublished manuscript.

Holloran, J. *Understanding Homosexual Persons: Straight Answers from Gays.* Hicksville, NY: Exposition Press, 1970. pp. 65-70.

Jones, A.B.S. *Volunteers' Resistance to Working with Minorities and Addicts.* Washington, DC: Whitman-Walker Clinic, 1988.

Jones, A.B.S., and Izzo, J.A. *Share a Needle and You Share AIDS.* Washington, DC: Whitman-Walker Clinic, 1988. 46 pp.

Morales, E.S., and Graves, M.A. *Substance Abuse: Patterns and Barriers to Treatment for Gay Men & Lesbians in San Francisco.* San Francisco: San Francisco Department of Public Health, 1988.

National Academy of Sciences. *Confronting AIDS: Directions for Public Health, Health Care, and Research.* Institute of Medicine, National Academy of Sciences. Washington, DC: National Academy Press, 1986.

Raymond, J.G. *The Transsexual Empire: The Making of the She-Male.* Boston: Beacon Press, 1979. pp. 101-113.

Tsang, D. *The Age Taboo.* Boston, MA: Alyson Publishing, 1981.

Weathers, B. *Alcoholism & the Lesbian Community.* Washington, DC: Whitman-Walker Clinic, 1981. 12 pp.

Weinberg, M., and Williams, C. *Male Homosexuals, Their Problems and Adaptations.* New York City: Oxford University Press, 1974.

Wolff, C. *Bisexuality: A Study.* New York: Quartet Books, 1977. pp. 93-98.

Wooden, W., and Parker, J. *Men Behind Bars: Sexual Exploitation in Prison.* New York: Plenum Press, 1982. 264 pp.

Ziebold, T.O., and Mongeon, J.E. *Ways to Gay Sobriety.* Washington, DC: Whitman-Walker Clinic, 1980.

ACKNOWLEDGMENTS

The contributions of Joseph A. Izzo, M.A., M.S.W., Health Educator, and Claire Quigley, C.A.D.C., Director of Alcohol and Substance Abuse Services, Whitman-Walker Clinic, are acknowledged.

AUTHOR

A. Billy S. Jones, M.S.W.
Health Educator, Counselor, and Trainer
Assistant Director, Sunnye Sherman AIDS
    Education Services
Whitman-Walker Clinic
Suite 141
1407 S Street, N.W.
Washington, DC 20009

Risk Behavior of Intravenous Cocaine Users: Implications for Intervention

Dale D. Chitwood, Clyde B. McCoy, and Mary Comerford

INTRODUCTION

The primary aim of this chapter is to discuss specific characteristics of intravenous (IV) cocaine use, which are relevant for programs to reduce risk behavior for human immunodeficiency virus (HIV-1) transmission and exposure.

Two phenomena, the acquired immunodeficiency syndrome (AIDS) epidemic and IV cocaine use, have enormous consequences for IV drug users (IVDUs). The AIDS epidemic is the most consequential event of the 1980s and will continue to affect IVDUs for the foreseeable future (Des Jarlais and Friedman 1987; Ginzburg et al. 1985; Ginzburg 1988; Morgan and Curran 1988). The increasing prevalence of cocaine use among IVDUs also is important (Grabowski 1984; Kozel and Adams 1985), but has been overshadowed by the impact of AIDS. Although each phenomenon would have occurred in the absence of the other, these two major events effect each other. As the data presented in this chapter illustrate, the IV use of cocaine contributes to the risk behaviors for exposure to HIV-1 among many IVDUs, while at the same time an awareness of AIDS is leading some individuals who inject cocaine to change their needle/syringe and sexual behaviors.

PREVALENCE OF HIV-1

The use of cocaine has been found to be associated with serostatus for antibodies to HIV-1. Chaisson et al. (1988) have reported that IVDUs who use cocaine frequently are more likely to be positive for HIV-1 than other IVDUs. In Miami, 255 IV cocaine users in drug treatment who had injected cocaine during the past 12 months were twice as likely (20.8 percent) to test positive for antibodies to HIV-1

120

as were 222 persons who had injected opiates only (9.5 percent). Among the 255 IV cocaine users, 56 clients who injected only cocaine were as likely to test positive (24.5 percent) as were the 199 IV users who had injected cocaine and opiates (19.8 percent).

METHODOLOGY

Two types of information are presented in this chapter that deal with the issues of AIDS prevention for IV cocaine users.

First, it is useful to have an understanding of the nature of the IV use of cocaine as it existed when IV cocaine users were being exposed to HIV but prior to anyone, including IV cocaine users, even suspecting that AIDS existed. In order to do this, data are reported from an investigation of patterns of cocaine use that were occurring in the late 1970s and early 1980s. Between April 1980 and June 1981 a structured interview was administered to 75 IV cocaine users who were a subgroup of 170 cocaine users in south Florida (Chitwood 1985). A subsample of those IV cocaine users also provided an open-ended interview, which was taped and transcribed (Morningstar and Chitwood 1984). These data are reported to document characteristics of IV cocaine use that are believed to increase risk behavior for exposure to HIV-1, as well as to identify characteristics that should be considered in prevention efforts.

A second data source was selected to document specific risk behaviors that currently are practiced by IV cocaine users and identify changes in these behaviors that users report have occurred as a result of their efforts to avoid AIDS. The risk behavior data reported here are baseline data from a longitudinal epidemiologic investigation of HIV-1 infection among IVDUs in South Florida. Between June 1987 and July 1988, 722 IVDUs in drug treatment programs in south Florida were interviewed about their drug use, needle/syringe (works) behavior, and sexual behavior and were tested for antibodies to HIV-1. Risk behavior data were reported for 255 triethnic men and women who were active IV cocaine users. Of the 255, 199 participants had injected cocaine and opiates in the year prior to baseline interview, either simultaneously, as speedball (a mixture of cocaine and an opiate, usually heroin), or, less often, serially. An additional 56 had injected only cocaine.

The majority of these 255 IV cocaine users were non-Hispanic white (61.2 percent), while 26.7 percent were non-Hispanic black and 11.0 percent were Hispanic. Three persons (1.1 percent) were American

Indian or Oriental. Two-thirds (67.8 percent) of all respondents were male.

There were no ethnic or gender differences between those who injected only cocaine and others who injected both cocaine and opiates. Approximately four out of every five non-Hispanic white (76.6 percent), non-Hispanic black (83.9 percent), and Hispanic (82.1 percent) users injected both cocaine and opiates. Similarly, 79.2 percent of the men and 75.6 percent of the women injected cocaine and opiates.

FINDINGS

The findings reported in this chapter are divided into three distinct sections.

First, this chapter discusses specific characteristics of the IV use of cocaine as determined from both structured interview schedules that contained extensive items concerning drug history, IV behavior, and sexual behavior, and open-ended interviews with cocaine users about their views of the nature of IV cocaine use. The purpose of this discussion is to identify elements of IV cocaine use that predispose users to engage in high-risk behavior.

Second, specific high-risk behaviors of current IV cocaine users are reported for the purpose of documenting high-risk behaviors that risk reduction programs must target.

Third, specific changes in high-risk behaviors that IV cocaine users said they initiated without involvement in a risk reduction program are presented to illustrate areas where interventions might be effective.

Characteristics That Potentiate High-Risk Behavior

IV cocaine use was studied in the early 1980s as part of a comprehensive investigation of the patterns of cocaine use in south Florida (Morningstar and Chitwood 1984; Chitwood and Morningstar 1985). Most of the 75 IV cocaine users in that study reported they craved increasing quantities of cocaine but had inadequate resources to fulfill that desire. Approximately two-thirds (68.0 percent) of the 75 IV cocaine users who participated in that study said they were obsessed with the desire for cocaine. At the time of the interview, a majority (61.3 percent) were using cocaine more frequently than they had in their initial year of use (Chitwood 1985). Three-fourths (72.0 percent) had no personal limit on the amount of money they spent for cocaine--if funds were available. Not surprisingly, 81.3 percent of these IV cocaine users reported that they had money problems as a consequence of their cocaine use.

Many IV cocaine users (61.3 percent) reported that they always craved cocaine when it was present, and 4 out of 10 (44.0 percent) never had refused cocaine, regardless of the setting and circumstances under which it was offered to them.

When cocaine users were asked what patterns of cocaine use they had observed, their own perceptions of themselves supported a similar typology of use (Morningstar and Chitwood 1984). Cocaine users described several traits of IV cocaine use behavior that would increase the likelihood that IV cocaine users might engage in high-risk injection or sexual behaviors. IV cocaine users often were reported to have an "addictive predisposition," to be obsessed with obtaining cocaine they could not afford, and not to care what they did to obtain cocaine. Furthermore, many IV cocaine users were perceived by cocaine users as antisocial persons who would "rip off" others for drugs (Morningstar and Chitwood 1984.)

These traits indicate that IV cocaine use often becomes uncontrolled behavior, and, when cocaine is available under high-risk conditions, many users are likely to engage in those behaviors to obtain cocaine.

This is borne out in self-report data about specific behaviors in which those IV cocaine users engaged to obtain cocaine. For example, 46.6 percent reported that they had engaged in either prostitution or pimping to obtain money for cocaine. A similar percentage (45.3 percent) reported they traded sexual favors for cocaine. When differences between cocaine acquisition methods of men and women were observed, men tended to be more aggressive and women to be more manipulative (Morningstar and Chitwood 1987). Several women reported they used sex to get cocaine from men, while men frequently said they used cocaine to entice women to have sex with them. Regardless of which perspective is more accurate, it is clear that high-risk sexual behavior often is bartered for cocaine. One additional observation is of major consequence. Most men and women were introduced to cocaine use by male friends or spouses. Indeed, the cocaine dealing system tends to be male dominated, and a majority of women often are dependent upon men for their cocaine source. Consequently, women may be more likely, when sharing works, to shoot after a male partner, a behavior that puts women at risk for HIV-1 exposure when works remain uncleaned.

In summary, several aspects of IV cocaine use lead to high-risk behavior for exposure to HIV-1: obsessive behavior, lack of funds to obtain cocaine, strong craving in the presence of cocaine, never refusing cocaine regardless of setting, use of cocaine with strangers, having sex to get cocaine or using cocaine to obtain a casual sexual partner, and shooting after others upon whom one is dependent for cocaine.

Most of these traits were present in a plurality, often the majority, of study participants who were injecting cocaine in the early 1980s, before AIDS had been detected/identified.

Current Risk Behaviors for HIV-1

Current risk behaviors of cocaine users were ascertained by asking 255 persons enrolled in drug treatment programs who had injected cocaine during the prior year several questions about their injection and sexual behaviors during the 12 months prior to their interview. Three general patterns of IV cocaine use were reported by this study sample:

(1)   injection of cocaine only;

(2)   injection of cocaine and an opiate simultaneously, as speedball; and

(3)   injection of cocaine and opiates serially.

Two methods used to prepare cocaine for injection increase the risk of using a dirty needle and thus the risk of exposure to HIV-1. The first method has been reported by cocaine users who do not inject opiates. Some persons who inject cocaine reported that they pool funds with others and together prepare several syringes before they begin their run. These works may or may not be sterile at this juncture. Once the run or binge begins, they continue to reuse works indiscriminately until the cocaine supply is exhausted. A second high-risk procedure often is used to prepare speedball—a mixture of an opiate (usually heroin) and cocaine, a combination which has been used for decades (O'Donnell and Ball 1966). This method involves drawing the opiate into one syringe and the cocaine into a second syringe and mixing the contents between the two syringes. The procedure is as follows: in one cooker, an opiate is placed into solution by heating ("cooking"). In a second cooker, cocaine is stirred (not cooked) into solution. (A variation is to cold-shake cocaine and water in a syringe instead of mixing in a cooker.) These liquids are drawn into separate syringes and then mixed from syringe to syringe. This involves removing the needle from one syringe and injecting the contents of the other syringe into the needleless syringe. Then the process is reversed. This results in two syringes filled with speedball. If either syringe is unsterile, both syringes will become contaminated. The risk of exposure is heightened when unsterile syringes from shooting galleries are used, exposing the two users to the contaminants of both syringes.

The percentage of IV cocaine users who engaged in high-risk behaviors in the year prior to interview is presented in table 1. Information is presented for persons who inject cocaine only and for others who inject both cocaine and opiates.

The first portion of table 1 contains information about high-risk injection behaviors. Note that in most instances persons who inject cocaine alone are somewhat less likely to have practiced these behaviors than those who inject cocaine and opiates. The majority (56.9 percent) of all respondents had injected cocaine on an average of at least once per day. Eighty percent booted when they were injecting drugs. Booting involves the aspiration of venous blood into the syringe to mix the drug solution with the blood. This mixed solution then is injected into the vein. This process increases the likelihood that contaminants in the syringe would be injected into the user.

High-risk sharing of drug paraphernalia also was practiced by most respondents. Seven out of ten (70.6 percent) had shared cookers and 71.8 percent had shared works (needle/syringe combinations) at some time during the last year. About one-fourth (25.9 percent) also had used works of a shooting gallery during that time period.

Data in table 1 also indicate the extent of high-risk sexual behavior among IV cocaine users. No differences were found between those who inject only cocaine and other IV cocaine users. Almost all respondents (91.0 percent) had been sexually active in the past year.

Approximately half (51.4 percent) had one or more sexual partners who also had a history of IV drug use, while 63.1 percent reported they had a sexual partner(s) who had not injected drugs.

TABLE 1. *Proportion engaged in risk behaviors in last 12 months*

	Cocaine Only Users (n=56) %	Cocaine and Opiate Users (n=199) %	Between-Group Difference p-value	All Cocaine Users (n=255) %
Injection Behavior				
Injected at least daily	41.1	61.3	<.01	58.0
Booted	67.9	83.4	<.05	80.0
Shared cooker	51.8	75.9	<.001	70.6
Shared works	58.9	75.4	<.05	71.8
Shared works at shooting gallery	16.1	28.6	n.s.	25.9
Sexual Behavior				
Sexually active	91.1	91.0	n.s.	91.0
IV sexual partner(s)	53.6	50.8	n.s.	51.4
Other sexual partner(s)	57.1	64.9	n.s.	63.1
Never use condom	76.8	69.8	n.s.	71.4
Use condom at least 50% of time	10.7	10.1	n.s.	10.2

Condoms seldom were used by any of the study respondents or their sexual partners. Only 28.6 percent of the participants reported any condom use during sexual activity in the last year, and only 1 in 10 (10.2 percent) used a condom at least 50 percent of the time they engaged in sexual activity.

Changes in Risk Behavior

It does appear that IV cocaine users are willing to make behavioral changes to reduce their risk of AIDS. Of the 255 respondents in treatment who reported some IV cocaine use in the past year, 179 (70.2 percent) reported that they had changed some high-risk behavior to reduce the risk of AIDS. These changes in risk behavior were elicited at baseline before respondents had been tested for antibodies to HIV-1. Table 2 shows the reported changes made by these IV cocaine users.

TABLE 2. *Proportion reporting behavior changes to reduce risk of AIDS*

Behavior Change	Cocaine Only Users (n=56) %	Cocaine and Opiate Users (n=199) %	Between- Group Difference p-value	All Cocaine Users (n=255) %
Any behavior change	67.9	70.9	n.s.	70.2
Quit shooting drugs	8.9	4.0	n.s.	5.1
Quit sharing needles	16.1	21.1	n.s.	20.0
Shared needles less frequently	12.5	24.1	n.s.	21.6
Cleaned needles with bleach or alcohol	12.5	13.6	n.s.	13.3
Reduced number of sexual partners	25.0	24.6	n.s.	24.7
Reduced number of casual sexual encounters	12.5	11.6	n.s.	11.8
Used condoms more frequently	8.9	11.6	n.s.	11.0

While only 5.1 percent of the respondents reported that they had ceased all IV drug use, an additional 20 percent said that they had stopped sharing needles. Another 21.6 percent indicated that they shared needles less frequently. About 1 out of 10 (13.3 percent) stated they had begun cleaning works with bleach or alcohol.

Some respondents also reported changes in sexual behavior. One quarter (24.7 percent) had reduced the number of sexual partners during the preceding year, and 11.8 percent had reduced the number of casual sexual encounters. More frequent use of condoms was reported by 11.0 percent of these IV cocaine users.

While these data were self-reported and are not verifiable independently, they do indicate that IV cocaine users are aware of the need for behavior changes and are willing to attempt making them. In addition, none of these changes were initiated as part of any formal intervention program designed to elicit behavior changes. It appears that some IV cocaine users are aware of the role of some high-risk behaviors in the transmission of HIV-1 and are sufficiently concerned to attempt to change their high-risk needle use and sexual behaviors. These data are consistent with reports that IVDUs are willing to make behavior changes to reduce the risk of AIDS (Chaisson et al. 1987; Friedman et al. 1986).

All respondents also were asked why they changed their works. Most (71.0 percent) said they did so because the works became dull or ceased to operate properly. Only three (1.2 percent) changed works because of fear of AIDS, while an additional 7.1 percent changed works to avoid hepatitis and other common infections.

DISCUSSION

Three basic observations are evident from these data. First of all, the IV use of cocaine, because of the compulsive behavior that often accompanies use, frequently results in injection and/or sexual behavior that places that person at high risk for exposure to HIV-1. Because of this, it is essential that risk behavior reduction programs be developed for cocaine users.

Second, the data suggest that intervention will have to occur on various levels of prevention. The fact that 7 out of 10 IV cocaine users (70.2 percent) report some self-initiated efforts to reduce risk behavior indicates that intervention has the potential to succeed.

In fact, many cocaine users go through periods when they voluntarily cease cocaine use (Chitwood 1985). However, it would be naive to develop an intervention that assumed cessation of high-risk behaviors, e.g., IV cocaine use, would be achievable in all instances. Secondary prevention goals with specific intervention strategies, e.g., not sharing drug paraphernalia, cleaning works, using condoms during sexual activity, must be part of risk reduction programs, because a proportion of users will continue to inject cocaine.

In the absence of effective medical treatment and vaccines, risk reduction programs must be implemented to restrain the epidemic. The general objectives of these programs should be to stop or at least reduce (1) the use of drugs, (2) the IV use of drugs, and (3) the sharing of needles/syringe (works). In addition, for those who will not stop sharing works, emphasis must be placed on the proper method to sterilize used works before sharing. Similarly, efforts must be targeted to increase the practice of safer sex behaviors, such as the use of condoms, and to avoid pregnancy if HIV-1 antibody positive. The specific goals of each program will vary according to the composition of the population selected for intervention.

Third, the optimal intervention package would be enhanced if it could incorporate the following six program elements.

(1) Prevention programs must be aimed at specific ethnic groups if the intervention is to be most effective. Cocaine users are found among several ethnic groups. Culturally specific characteristics of the ethnic communities being targeted, e.g., an emphasis on the role of the family among Hispanic cocaine users (Marin 1988), must be developed and implemented within the prevention program.

(2) Issues of gender must be acknowledged and incorporated into the intervention. Specific intervention programs or program components must be developed for women, many of whom are dependent upon men not only for cocaine but for other economic and security needs as well. Programs for women will have to grapple with dependency/empowerment needs while recognizing that empowerment efforts may bring new pressures upon women who inject cocaine (Treasure and Liao 1982).

(3) Intervention programs must acknowledge the compulsive nature of cocaine. The ideal solution is to succeed in having the user cease cocaine use. However, it is essential to realize that, in those instances where cessation does not occur, there is an enormous compulsion to inject cocaine regardless of the setting for use. Many persons who use cocaine intravenously report a number of personal characteristics that increase the likelihood that they will engage in high-risk behavior. These include obsession with acquiring cocaine, frequent inability to afford

cocaine, craving cocaine when it is present, never refusing cocaine regardless of the setting or conditions for the acquisition of cocaine, shooting after another person with a dirty needle, exchanging sex for cocaine or funds to purchase cocaine.

Cocaine use has increased among methadone maintenance clients over the last 10 years, and IV use is a major route of ingestion among these clients (Kosten et al. 1987). Although methadone programs have been successful in reducing IV use (Ball et al. 1988), it is essential that intervention programs be implemented in methadone maintenance clinics. While the primary goal of the treatment program is the complete cessation of all drug use, including cocaine use, education and counseling in HIV transmission and prevention are necessary to reach clients who will not stop injecting cocaine.

Many persons who inject cocaine frequently engage in high-risk drug use behavior, including sharing cookers and works and using works from a shooting gallery. In these circumstances, users are likely to use dirty works if new ones or bleach and water to clean works are not readily available or if they do not know how to clean those works. Risk reduction programs must train IV cocaine users to clean works and to develop strategies for making the cleaning process an integral part of use. Users must be convinced that they should no longer use shooting galleries. In a parallel action, individuals who operate shooting galleries are in a strong position to reduce the risk for exposure to HIV-1. These individuals, if they learn how to clean works and become convinced that new or clean works are best for business, could reduce the potential for exposure by cleaning all works after each use.

(4) Cocaine users must shift their purpose for cleaning needles from rinsing in water to prevent the clogging of the needle/syringe to using bleach and water to destroy HIV-1 before the works are shared. This requires the development of strategies to convince the active drug user to integrate the sterilization of works into the fabric of IV drug use behavior.

(5) Intervention programs also must focus on high-risk sexual behavior. Many IV cocaine users engage in high-risk sexual behavior such as having multiple partners and partners who also inject drugs. These sexually active respondents seldom use

condoms. The exchange of sex for money or cocaine is common and, again, few use protection in the form of condoms. Nearly two-thirds of the 255 respondents interviewed in 1987 and 1988 had sexual partners who had never injected drugs. Several of those sexual partners will be exposed to HIV-1 infection from their partners who do inject drugs. Programs must be prepared to deal with the difficult issues of how an IV cocaine user who tests positive for antibodies to HIV-1 can tell his or her sexual partner. Provision should be made for counseling the IV user and the sexual partner together. Because the likelihood exists that such a revelation will disrupt/destroy some relationships, staff must be prepared to deal with this eventuality.

(6) Followup should be part of a comprehensive intervention. The risk behavior of many cocaine users will vary considerably over time. Behavioral changes that are achieved at the time of the initial intervention need to be reinforced over time.

The need to intervene to stop the spread of HIV-1 is so great that risk reduction programs must be implemented immediately. Unfortunately, most risk reduction programs are in their embryonic phases and definitive effective methods of intervention are only beginning to emerge. Therefore, it is essential that the effectiveness of these programs be evaluated simultaneously with the development of the programs. The results of these evaluations will enable interventionists to refine programs to improve their effectiveness.

REFERENCES

Ball, J.C.; Lange, W.R.; Myers, C.P.; and Friedman, S.R. Reducing the risk of AIDS through methadone maintenance treatment. *J Health Soc Behav* 29:214-226, 1988.

Chaisson, R.E.; Moss, A.R.; Onishi, R.; Osmond, D.D.; and Carlson, S.R. Human immunodeficiency virus infection in heterosexual intravenous drug users in San Francisco. *Am J Public Health* 77:169-172, 1987.

Chaisson, R.E.; Osmmond, P.; Bacchetti, B.; et al. Cocaine, race and HIV infection in IV drug users (abstract). Presented at the Fourth International Conference on AIDS, Stockholm, June 1988.

Chitwood, D.D. Patterns and consequences of cocaine use. In: Kozel, N.J., and Adams, E.H., eds. *Cocaine Use in America: Epidemiological and Clinical Perspectives*. National Institute on Drug Abuse Research Monograph 61. DHHS Pub. No. (ADM)85-1414. Washington, DC: Supt. of Docs., U.S. Govt. Print. Off. 1985, pp. 111-129.

Chitwood, D.D., and Morningstar, P.C. Factors which differentiate cocaine users in treatment from non-treatment users. *Int J Addict* 20:449-459, 1985.

Des Jarlais, D.C., and Friedman, S.R. HIV infection among intravenous drug users: Epidemiology and risk reduction. *AIDS Int J* 1:67-76, 1987.

Friedman, S.R.; Des Jarlais, D.C.; and Sotheran, J.L. AIDS health education for intravenous drug users. *Health Educ Q* 13:268-272, 1986.

Ginzburg, H.M. Acquired immune deficiency syndrome (AIDS) and drug abuse. In: Galea, R.P.; Lewis, B.S.; and Baker, L.A., eds. *AIDS and IV Drug Abusers*. Owings Mills, MD: National Health Publishing, 1988. pp. 61-74.

Ginzburg, H.M.; Weiss, S.H.; MacDonald, M.G.; and Hubbard, R.L. HTLV-III exposure among drug users. *Ca Res* 45:4605s-4608s, 1985.

Grabowski, J., ed. *Cocaine: Pharmacology, Effects, and Treatment of Abuse*. National Institute on Drug Abuse Research Monograph 50. DHHS Pub. No. (ADM)84-1326. Washington, DC: Supt. of Docs., U.S. Govt. Print. Off., 1984. pp. 1-14.

Kosten, T.R.; Schumann, B.; Wright, D.; Carney, M.K.; and Garvin, F.H. A preliminary study of desipramine in the treatment of cocaine abuse in methadone maintenance patients. *J Clin Psychiatry* 48:442-444, 1987.

Kozel, N.J., and Adams, E.H., eds. *Cocaine Use in America: Epidemiologic and Clinical Inspections*. National Institute on Drug Abuse Research Monograph 61. DHHS Pub. No. (ADM)85-1414. Washington DC: Supt. of Docs., U.S. Govt. Print. Off., 1985. 129 pp.

Marin, G. AIDS prevention issues among Hispanics. Paper presented at the American Psychological Association, Atlanta, Georgia, August 1988.

Morgan, W.M., and Curran, J.W. Acquired immunodeficiency syndrome: Current and future trends. In: Galea, R.P.; Lewis, B.F.; and Baker, L.A., eds. *AIDS and IV Drug Abusers*. Owings Mills, MD: National Health Publishing, 1988. pp. 267-280.

Morningstar, P.J., and Chitwood, D.D. Cocaine users view of themselves. Implicit behavior theory in context. *Human Organization* 43:307-318, 1984.

Morningstar, P.J., and Chitwood, D.D. How women and men get cocaine: Sex-role stereotypes and acquisition patterns. *J Psychoactive Drugs* 19:135-142, 1987.

O'Donnell, J.A., and Ball, J.C., eds. *Narcotic Addiction*. New York: Harper & Row, 1966. p. 4.

Treasure, K.G., and Liao, H. Survival skills training for drug dependent women. In: Reed, B.G.; Beschner, J.M.; and Mondanaro, J., eds. *Treatment Services for Drug Dependent Women*. Vol. II. National Institute on Drug Abuse. DHHS Pub. No. (ADM)82-1219. Washington, DC: Supt. of Docs., U.S. Govt. Print. Off., 1982. pp. 137-158.

AUTHORS

Dale D. Chitwood, Ph.D.
Associate Professor
Clyde B. McCoy, Ph.D.
Professor
Mary Comerford, M.S.P.H.
Research Associate

Department of Oncology
Division of Cancer Control
University of Miami School of Medicine
Room 309
1550 N.W. 10th Avenue
Miami, FL 33136

An Ethnographic Approach to Understanding HIV High-Risk Behaviors: Prostitution and Drug Abuse

Michele G. Shedlin

INTRODUCTION

Our gaps in knowledge about the acquired immunodeficiency syndrome (AIDS) epidemic and the role of prostitution in human immunodeficiency virus (HIV) transmission make it unwise to assume that we are sufficiently informed about "the oldest profession" as it is practiced in our inner cities today. The high-risk behaviors involved in the sale of recreational sex, and the use of intravenous (IV) drugs (as both cause and consequence of prostitution) need to be studied further if we are to develop effective prevention strategies. These behaviors require research "in the field," both at the level of the individual and the "community" as defined by its cultures of drug use and prostitution.

If we are to achieve behavioral change in these communities and develop mechanisms that will sustain this change, we must attempt to understand existing behaviors. Quantitative data alone, however important in identifying the outcomes of behavior, do not provide us with an understanding of how, when, where, or why they occur. Surveys that rely upon predetermined sets of variables do not permit discovery and exploration. Moreover, survey research assumes that "outsiders" as interviewers will be recording truths from one-time contacts with individuals whose very survival depends upon lies, deception, and the expert manipulation of "outsiders." Rather, painstaking field research is necessary to provide the data needed for the microanalysis of high-risk behaviors common to communities implicated in HIV transmission.

As we know, an institutionally based program which reaches out into the community is not the same as a community-based approach which requires far greater knowledge of the community itself for the design and implementation of interventions. An emphasis on qualitative research, combined with the utilization of quantitative data, is important in identifying not only the high-risk behaviors of these communities, but also the information crucial to the design of appropriate and acceptable programs. This information may include:

- perceived community needs;

- the cultural (and subcultural) factors that influence the acceptability and utilization of information and services;

- formal and informal communication networks;

- existing beliefs and knowledge that determine or influence behavior;

- the identification of potential program resources; and

- the identification of existing or potential obstacles in service delivery and/or the acceptance and utilization of services.

The data presented here represent a part of the qualitative research carried out with prostitutes in New York City and Bridgeport, Connecticut, and focus upon the beliefs and behaviors that place them at risk for HIV infection and transmission.

BACKGROUND OF THE RESEARCH

In 1986, I was asked to assist with a program that involved working with street prostitutes in New York City. Although my objectives were oriented toward social service rather than research, a colleague at the Centers for Disease Control (CDC) convinced me to begin an analytical harvesting of my experience and observations with this population. In April 1987, I began work in Bridgeport, the largest of Connecticut's cities, to develop a model for reaching prostitutes with AIDS prevention education. The baseline research for developing this program involved semistructured, in-depth, and informal conversational interviews with street prostitutes and call girls. Interviews were also carried out with substance abuse treatment professionals, topless-bar owners, city health officials, politicians, clients of prostitutes, and businessmen who regularly provide prostitutes to their clients.

This paper does not attempt to generalize the data presented on perceptions, attitudes, and behaviors to all prostitutes. Nor is it an exhaustive treatment of the sex-related attitudes and behaviors of prostitute populations in Bridgeport or New York City. The objective of this paper is to illustrate the type of qualitative data that can be useful in developing and directing intervention strategies and educational materials.

It should be noted that all prostitutes interviewed in Bridgeport were currently, or had been, IV drug abusers, and most were recruited through a local methadone maintenance program. While many of those in methadone treatment continue to abuse drugs, they do not produce the "dirty" urines that would cause them to be dropped from the program. Thus, the women interviewed were still using some type of drug and prostituting at the time of the interview.

In addition to a year of informal conversational interviews and observation on the street and in a methadone clinic, over 30 hours of open-ended, semistructured interviews with 15 prostitutes were carried out. I stressed the confidentiality of the information, explained the objectives of the data collection (project development), and made it very clear, for my own protection and theirs, that I did not want information about the providers of drugs or their locations. I attempted to obtain descriptive information specific to the practice of prostitution in the area to assist in the design of the street prostitution project, as well as more in-depth information concerning attitudes, beliefs, and behaviors relating to the sale of recreational sex. Although everyone in the drug treatment program from which I recruited most of the interviewees had to permit HIV testing as a prerequisite for treatment admission, I never asked questions about test results. In almost every case, however, results were volunteered, both positive and negative.

In order to communicate appropriately, one area stressed in the interview was language. Prostitutes call themselves "working girls," and "business girls"; their clients are "dates" or, less frequently, "johns." The terms "hooker" and "trick" are seen as derogatory. Condoms are most frequently called "rubbers"; however, some girls call them "condos." Oral sex is referred to as a "B.J." (blow job), and "half and half" means oral and vaginal sex. Anal sex is referred to as "greeking," "annual intercourse," and "up the dirt road." Their "old man" is usually a pimp, the other women in his "stable" are known to each other as "wives-in-law." "On the stroll" expresses the street girls' daily (or nightly) activity. Women who do not "work" are "straight."

Drug-related vocabulary also pervades their speech. Drug parapher-nalia are known as "works"; needles are "spikes"; a "hitter" is some-one who is paid to inject; a "cooker" is a bottle cap or anything used to "melt dope"; and "copping" or "scoring" mean buying drugs. You don't use drugs, you "do drugs," and everyone tries to hide the "tracks" on their bodies, which testify to IV drug use.

CHARACTERISTICS OF THE PROSTITUTES

"Prostitute" is not a homogeneous category. While Sydney Biddle Barrows, the "Mayflower Madam," recruited nursing students, strug-gling actresses, and divorcing housewives for her call service, most prostitutes are not the middle-class and upper middle-class women described by her or the movie "Working Girls" (produced by Miramax Films in 1986). These women occupy a high rung in the hierarchy of prostitution. The better escort or call services recruit the younger, prettier, better educated women who are less frequently drug addicted (many agencies forbid drug use) and are more often working for fast money than to support a habit or a pimp. The New York Police Department estimates that there are several hundred prostitute loca-tions that can call on between 50 and 150 girls from as far away as Rhode Island. Bridgeport has numerous call/escort services; however, most are small-scale operations.

Topless bars and massage parlors occupy the next level of this hier-archy. The girls generally obtain customers through these businesses, paying a percentage of their earnings to the owners, or being paid directly by the owners for their sexual services. The dancers tend to change bars and areas frequently, as their principal draw is a "new commodity." Interestingly, many potential johns expect the "exotic dancer" to maintain the charade that she is only a dancer and not a prostitute. Even though he may "convince" her to have sex and pay her for her services, he rationalizes that he has "made it" with a dancer. This also holds for dancer/strippers at stag parties, who are raffled off at the end of the evening. They are expected to have some form of sex with at least one guest for the total fee, but are not hired as prostitutes. Street prostitutes, call girls, and johns dis-tinguish dancers from others who sell recreational sex.

"Street girls" occupy the bottom rung in the hierarchy; however, the individuals on the street represent a huge range in age, education,

137

ethnicity, drug involvement, and price. In New York City, a group of prostitutes with whom I worked in the midtown area were well-educated, well-dressed Canadian and midwestern women who charged fees usually reserved for call girls. They provided sexual services to Wall Street executives and wealthy tourists in a nearby hotel, turning over an average of $100,000 a year to their pimps.

At the bottom of the street scale are the throwaway children, unwanted by parents or family, who are put on the street by their pimps, usually very late at night, or the drug-addicted mother who works to support her children and her habit, not necessarily in that order.

With the exception of the middle-class moonlighter who is short on money and "getting by" by temporarily prostituting, there are some common denominators which psychologists and social service professionals have identified. Prostitutes tend to have been sexually abused or physically abused and/or neglected as children. Many were throwaway children. Another common factor, both cause and effect of their activities, is an overwhelming lack of ego, sense of self-worth, and perception of any alternative way of life. This characteristic is important in understanding their attitudes about sex, professionally and personally.

It is also important to recognize that many prostitutes are mothers. Whether wanted and loved, or unwanted and relinquished to the State or relatives, these women in reproductive age have borne, and are bearing children. Almost every prostitute interviewed had one or more children. Often, their only aspirations are for their children. Even the most strung-out addict, who cared nothing about her body or her future, expressed guilt and concern about her children. Prostitutes have reported that their greatest fear is that of being investigated by social service agencies and having their children taken away. This possibility was given as a reason for not utilizing city health services—the fear of officials learning of their prostitution and drug abuse and removing the children to foster homes. Some of the women in Bridgeport limit their prostitution to the daytime, not only to avoid the dangers of the street at night, but to be home when the children leave daycare or return from school.

The concern for their children, for the health and well-being of existing and future children, may be an important element in promoting behavioral change. It is important to take this into consideration in researching and designing programs.

Role of the Pimp

A question that is consistently asked is, "How does the pimp get and keep women who support him? What does he have?" The caricature of the tall, black, ostentatious character in a wide-brimmed hat and fancy car is indeed a reality of the street scene. Many pimps, however, are silent and low-key, black or white. They are, characteristically, excellent natural psychologists, able to recruit a young runaway in a bus station in less than 20 minutes. They promise love, security, protection . . . everything denied to the abused or throwaway child. Their keeping-power is said to be any combination of fear, drugs, affection, sexual attention, and the fathering and control of a prostitute's children.

As Flexner reported in 1914:

> The tie is easy to describe, difficult to understand . . . .
> One is thrown back for an adequate explanation on the
> fundamental fact of the sex relation. The woman has no
> attachment whatsoever with her stream of casual
> customers, but the pimp belongs to her. (Flexner 1914,
> p. 32)

The women who belong to a pimp vie for his attention and sexual favors, competing to be his "main woman." He uses this competition, favoring the one who brings in the most money. I have heard of prostitutes who have taken years of dreadful abuse; others who have left pimps to work independently elsewhere; and still others who have married their pimps—often the fathers of their children. "A girl likes that control if she's been an outcast," said one of my informants. "To you it's abuse, to us he cares enough to beat her." Women who are controlled by pimps are typically difficult to reach. Some can be contacted only when the pimp is not around and then with great care, because contact could endanger the prostitute as well as the health care or social service worker. The Salvation Army has a mobile canteen that circulates in New York City late at night, serving coffee to the "girls" and thus contacting many who are otherwise not reachable, since the pimps are reluctant to interfere with "the Church" (Major Elizabeth Baker, personal communication). Many prostitutes will protect the social service street workers by ignoring or otherwise warning them when the pimp is around. The young children are the hardest to reach as they are constantly watched by their pimps.

Perceived Roles of the Prostitute

The prostitutes interviewed perceived their most important sexual function as providing what other women, "straight women," do not like or refuse to provide. Biddle Barrows states that a call girl is a woman who "knows how to satisfy certain needs that a man has, and who, at least professionally, accepts the very kind of behavior that other women in his life persist in regarding as amoral or a sign of weakness." (Biddle Barrows 1986, p. 174) Typically this "behavior" is oral sex, the most frequent service of the street prostitute and, usually, at least a part of the services provided by call girls. Clients interviewed also reported oral sex as their main activity with prostitutes. It is important to note, in considering oral sex as a risk factor in HIV transmission, that prostitutes are occasionally paid extra to swallow the ejaculate, and that they frequently have gum problems and oral lesions. Prostitutes also listed anal sex, bondage, and a range of fantasy behaviors as the services they provided that wives and girlfriends would not provide or that clients would not request of wives and girlfriends.

Prostitutes and their clients acknowledged that many johns need to degrade, humiliate, and otherwise control the prostitute during their sexual encounter. "The dirtier you are, the sluttier, the more they like it." "You gotta be a pure dog." "They pull hair, slap your face, talk dirty." "They have full control because they have money in their pocket and you on your knees . . . "; " . . . the turn-on is in control." For a woman with little or no self-esteem, this role is simply part of the job.

Biddle Barrows, as well as my informants, report that men use prostitutes because they can be sexually gratified without having to invest energy in a relationship, maintain an image, or please their partner. (Biddle Barrows 1986, p. 96) The street prostitutes interviewed saw their role as providing fast, easy, uncomplicated physical release and ego reinforcement in exchange for "cash up front." "I don't want the wining and dining routine," said one john. "Girls get too clingy."

Call girls, more typically than street prostitutes, provide companionship.

> Many men believe that a call girl is inherently worldly and that her sexual experience (real or imagined) somehow endows her with an added measure of wisdom. After all, she is supposed to be an expert at pleasing

men. And if she knows how to please me, the client reasons, she must therefore understand me. At the same time, he thinks, she can't possibly judge me. (Biddle Barrows 1986, p. 174)

However, even the street girls report "dates" that are exclusively conversation, usually concerning problems at home or work.

AREAS OF CONCERN

Intimacy vs. Sex

To elicit information concerning intimacy and sex, informants were asked to explain two quotes. One was taken from the movie "Working Girls": "I haven't cheated on my guy in 5 years," stated a call girl waiting for her next client. The second quote was one recorded during street work with a program in New York City. A very agitated prostitute was explaining her anger . . . a john had tried to kiss her . . . "and I said, 'if you wanna kiss, go home to your wife'."

Not cheating was explained in the following ways:

- It probably means whatever her guy doesn't want her to do, she doesn't do.

- She hasn't been mentally involved with what she was doing with the john.

- If she feels nothing, she hasn't betrayed him.

- No sexual gratification with the johns.

- It was for finance, not romance—that's not cheating.

- It would hurt him if she didn't get paid for it, if she did it for nothing and enjoyed it.

- She hasn't given her love to anyone . . . she hasn't made love.

- Emotionally she hasn't become attached—the only attachment is financial.

141

The distinction between the sale of recreational sex and emotional involvement was an easy one for my informants.

The second quote was designed to explore behavior and intimacy further. The significance of kissing elicited some of the most useful discussion, and questions about kissing usually generated introspection and thoughtful pauses in the interview. I was told that there were two cardinal rules that all prostitutes learn: (1) get your money first, and (2) don't kiss a john.

- You don't kiss, that's disgusting.

- Johns don't come out for that . . . it's not an emotional thing (sex) . . . strictly business.

- More older guys want to kiss . . . they're missing their wives.

- Listen, if you're a john, I will treat you as a john . . . if you want something simple like a kiss, go home . . . if you want something different than what you get at home, I can take care of that.

- She said he should go home because she didn't want her time wasted . . . he offended her.

- A kiss is different from sex . . . a way of communicating feelings.

- I won't kiss any guy . . . just something in me . . . it turns my stomach . . . a lot of girls won't kiss.

- You're faced up front with what you're doing . . . that's reality in the face . . . to a regular girl a blow job is disgusting.

- In jail they talk . . . what do you do . . . you kiss 'em? . . . Whoever taught you to be a whore?

- The most intimate thing you can really have.

- My husband says, 'I'm glad you do something with me that you won't do with anyone else . . . don't let anyone kiss you, it would destroy me.

- He wanted to kiss her maybe because he was getting emotionally involved.

Although the prostitutes interviewed differed in what they felt was the most "intimate" act (e.g., anal sex, vaginal intercourse, talking about personal things), there was an almost uniform distinction between kissing and sex. Although some stated that johns do not want to kiss, most felt it was the prostitute who would not do so. The exception seems to be the exotic dancer, who frequently deep kisses men in the audience, men who seem to have little reluctance to participate in this serial kissing. The dancer, as stated previously, however, is distinguished from a prostitute and may earn money just for kissing customers.

Power and Control

The subject of "control" in the dynamic between the prostitute and client arose spontaneously in many of the interviews and informal conversations. As discussed, prostitutes report that some clients need to debase them and assert control physically, sexually, and economically. A common perception is that the prostitute is controlled by a john, a pimp, a madam, and frequently a drug habit. While this may be all or partially true, there is another power dynamic inherent in the sale of recreational sex. As Biddle Barrows explains:

> Most girls assumed that the man would always be in control because he was paying for her company. This was the critical point, and I tried to make sure each girl understood that she was the one who was actually in control. 'It all depends on your attitude,' I explained, 'if you act like you're in control, you will be!' (Biddle Barrows 1986, p. 175)

I explored this subject of power and control by asking informants to explain a quote from "Working Girls": "You can control any man as long as you know what his sexual trip is."

- If you pick somebody up, you have to have a street rap in order to get what you want . . . you can find a way . . . certain things you can say to that john to get what you want . . . if he likes you, you use it . . .

- I made like I had feelings . . . they need that attention and affection.

- A girl takes control of which character inside him he will be with you.

143

- Nine out of ten times you can call what the situation turns out to be.

- When he's locked in on that (sex), he's just responding.

- In order for you to get paid, to be successful, you have to be in control.

- A man is vulnerable when he wants sex . . . If you are in control, you can make him do what you want.

- The man becomes the weaker sex once you get him in the bedroom . . . in bed she becomes the more powerful one as long as she knows what he's into . . .

- That's very true . . . if this man loves whipped cream, he says 'how much?' and your price is there . . . I always ask and they let me know . . . I'm in complete control as far as being able to manipulate him . . .

This last statement, interestingly, was made by the same woman who described the johns' need to degrade and control the prostitute.

Obviously, the fantasy and reality of power and control in the client/prostitute relationship is a complex issue, one that is influenced by many cultural, psychological, and situational factors. The importance of this issue for education and outreach is in identifying audiences and messages for the promotion of preventive behaviors. Can the prostitute insist on her client using a condom? How can she use her abilities to manipulate and control a situation to ensure her safety? How can we, as health professionals, utilize this information?

High-Risk "Tools of the Trade"

In discussing a "typical" day/night of drug use and prostitution with the prostitutes, they themselves mentioned a number of practices as "risky." "It's not just the needles," they said, "there's blood mixed in with the dope," "left in the 'cooker'", "blood can be in the cotton" (used to soak up drugs after cooking), "in the water." The practice of sharing needles and drugs sometimes signifies more than convenience and cost. Sharing drugs and works can be seen as a form of trust and street alliance. Sharing with the shooting gallery owner, his "tip," is an investment for the rainy day when they may be short the price of admission.

Another interesting practice relating to oral sex is the spitting of the ejaculate into rags or wads of tissues. These rags are then put back into their handbags for reuse. Meanwhile, the prostitutes take the money just earned, send a young boy to score their drugs, go to the shooting gallery, "hit" themselves or "get hit," and then use the same rag to wipe up excess blood from their body. The rags then go back into their handbags as they go back on the street.

The rag, cooker, and cotton are important details in understanding the risk factors in their behavior. Clearly, as differences in the prevalence of HIV illustrate, not all "communities" of prostitutes are doing the same thing the same way. The challenge of prevention research is to identify the components of their risk behaviors, which is more complex than simply identifying the use or nonuse of condoms or clean needles.

KNOWLEDGE, ATTITUDES, AND BEHAVIORS RELATING TO AIDS

The message that AIDS has no cure and that it is fatal <u>has</u> reached the streets. Prostitutes and their clients know that it is transmitted by sexual contact; addicts know that it is transmitted through shared needles. Yet unprotected sex continues to be sold, and "works" continue to be shared. There are many reasons for this, paramount among them being the nature of drug addiction. Poverty, addiction, low educational levels, a lack of self-esteem, hopelessness, and a lack of appropriate information and supporting services are also to blame.

The prostitutes report that AIDS and "crack" are the two major factors responsible for changes on the street. They perceive that older prostitutes are leaving the street because of their fear of AIDS and violence, and that continually younger women are taking their places because of addiction to "crack." "Some are young," said one veteran, "what a waste . . . they take a chance, getting arrested, getting AIDS . . . it's 'crack.'"

Many of my informants knew of someone who had died of AIDS; even more knew of companions with positive HIV test results. One prostitute who also lived by "boosting" (shoplifting), volunteered to work on an AIDS prevention education project shortly after learning that one of her friends had died. Most reported that those who died had "been on dope for years." One death discussed was that of "The Vampire." The name was given to a local shooting gallery owner who emptied leftover syringes into his veins, blood and all.

The association of IV drugs and AIDS is well known. "Everyone is so AIDS conscious. If they see tracks, they don't want you." "I lie, I say I've never touched a needle. I hide it." Business has improved in the underground sale of disposable needles used by diabetics, and some addicts have begun to check "cookers" and cotton (used for soaking up the liquified drug) for signs of blood. Prostitutes are now more careful about covering track marks so as not to scare off clients, but, I was told, a "girl" in need of a fix will not worry about dirty needles or using condoms.

One way of dealing with the fear of AIDS is to deny susceptibility to risk, or even to refuse information. "We don't want to be constantly reminded," I was chastised. "A lot of street girls are not afraid of AIDS." "I'm not spending all that money to buy those rubbers." They also warned me that prostitutes would not accept materials that said "AIDS" because someone seeing it would think they were reading the pamphlet or brochure because they already had AIDS.

Although I was told that AIDS can be transmitted by needles, open sores, saliva, "the rear if you have hemorrhoids," and semen, most of my informants were not really sure how AIDS could be transmitted. They asked if oral sex was safe. They asked about saliva. They asked about bleach, and were amazed to hear about Nonoxynol-9 lubricated condoms. It was my experience that information was welcome--at the appropriate time, and in an appropriate way.

When I asked what "safe sex" meant, I was told "There isn't any." Some said "abstinence"; others said "with rubbers." Although a few respondents volunteered that anal sex was probably a risky behavior, they said that johns asked for anal sex when they were afraid of herpes. (They are also paid more for anal sex.)

Condoms are more commonly used by call girls than by street girls. "Guys are very misinformed--they think they can have a thrill and get hard without a rubber and then only use it when they come." Few street girls use them in their main activity--oral sex. I was told that girls are in such a hurry to "get it over with" or "score" (buy drugs) that they don't care. They worry that if they insist on using a condom, the john will refuse and move up the street to another girl. The addict earning money for her next fix, or the prostitute threatened with a beating by her pimp if she does not bring in the required money, is not likely to risk losing a customer. They are also afraid that if they insist on the use of a condom, the john will think they already have AIDS.

146

HIV testing was generally seen to be punitive. Testing as a pre-requisite for the methadone program was enormously resented and resulted in a great deal of hostility toward the staff. Other sexually transmitted disease testing may also be associated with being arrested, at which time prostitutes are sometimes forced to accept tests. "When you get busted, the only blood test they give you is for GC [gonorrhea] not AIDS . . . and if they can't get a vein they say 'too bad, we're not gonna be involved in that!'"

Some prostitutes report that johns have actually asked to see HIV test results, and that "some madams want a note on them every 3 to 4 months from the health department!" "I go for tests all the time," said one informant, "especially now that I'm pregnant." One madam told me, "I don't want the responsibility for people dying . . . my girls are tested . . . I run a clean business."

Discussions with prostitutes who knew that they were HIV positive were heartrending. One of them seemed relieved to be able to share her trauma.

> I have been exposed to AIDS myself," she said casually. "I was in shock . . . it was two things at once, exposed to AIDS and pregnant at the same time. I associated it with death right away . . . In the past 6 months I've had a series of emotions, especially about AIDS . . . It doesn't affect you until it hits home . . . like rape . . . it really happens." She then added, "They told me over the phone . . . that's a bad way. They should have said 'come in' . . . if I had suicidal tendencies it would have had bad results . . . a working girl already feels bad . . ."

Another confided:

> I was giving up my 1½-year-old daughter . . . I felt I had nothing to offer my daughter because my aunt said "now you have AIDS, you're dying." I talked to a woman who runs Crossroads; she changed my outlook. Now I'm not signing papers . . . on my deathbed I will sign.

DESIGNING AN INTERVENTION MODEL

The objective of the research was to assist in the development of a model for AIDS prevention education for prostitutes. Thus, in addition to the questions concerning beliefs, knowledge, and behaviors relating to drug use and prostitution discussed here, the "girls" participated in guided discussions about AIDS prevention. The Bridgeport "girls" were not only willing, but eager to explore the "who," "when," "where," and "what" of program planning. They felt that they were the best category of outreach educator because they would have credibility and legitimacy with their peers. In addition, they felt they would have access to places and people not safe or "open" to "straight" individuals or health professionals (i.e., shooting galleries and topless bars). Their perceptions of needs for training, supervision, remuneration, and medical backup were explored over time, and a project proposal was prepared utilizing this research and an informal diagnosis of the city's available human and institutional resources.

One of the most interesting and productive aspects of this collaboration with the Bridgeport community of prostitutes was the development of a pamphlet on prevention exclusively for prostitutes. A group of three to five met regularly with me and with a graphic artist to design a pamphlet in a size that would fit in a handbag, select the content, decide on appropriate language, fine tune the graphics, and make decisions on the wording of a title which would attract, not discourage, its acceptance and consideration–*A Safety Guide for the Working Girl*. As the pamphlet became more of a reality, their sense of ownership and pride became clear, even to the point of requesting that their names be included on it as authors. For women whose overriding concern is anonymity, this was especially significant.

Obviously, the prostitutes themselves were an important resource in developing a community-based strategy. Their information and suggestions were used in conjunction with the information and advice of local health officials, politicians, and law enforcement personnel. Although the program and the educational pamphlet have yet to be evaluated, a program has begun, our data bank has increased, and the field research has been shared for others to consider and utilize.

Our challenge in identifying needs and resources, strengths and obstacles, questions and solutions, is formidable. I believe our best chance is to work closely with these communities to develop interventions that are subculturally acceptable and that will result in sustained behavioral change.

REFERENCES

Baker, Major Elizabeth, Salvation Army. Personal communication, 1987.

Biddle Barrows, S. *Mayflower Madam*. Arbor House, NY: Ivy Books, 1986. 291 pp.

Borden, L., and Kay, S. *Working Girls*. Miramax Films, 1986. (Film)

Flexner, A. *Prostitution in Europe*. 1914. Reprint. Montclair, NJ: Patterson Smith Publishing Company, 1969. 455 pp.

ACKNOWLEDGMENTS

Research was supported by Family Health International, Research Triangle Park, NC.

AUTHOR

Michele G. Shedlin, Ph.D.
Sociomedical Resource Associates, Inc.
Westport, CT 06880

The Role of Schools in Community-Based Approaches to Prevention of AIDS and Intravenous Drug Use

Lewayne D. Gilchrist

INTRODUCTION

During the last decade and a half, schools have increasingly become the focus for health promotion and disease prevention efforts aimed at both children and their families (Iverson and Kolbe 1983). The purpose of this chapter is to analyze the role that schools might play in community-based approaches to prevention of acquired immuno-deficiency syndrome (AIDS) and intravenous (IV) drug use. The analysis includes a summary of existing knowledge regarding human immunodeficiency virus (HIV) infection and AIDS prevention in school-age populations; consideration of factors that favor and that hinder effective AIDS prevention efforts in schools; review of documented experiences with health-related, school-based prevention programming; review of preliminary, anecdotal, and other less formally documented prevention programming in school settings; and, finally, suggestions for intervention models and future research initiatives.

HIV INFECTION AND AIDS PREVENTION FOR SCHOOL-AGE POPULATIONS

Less than 1 percent of total AIDS cases reported to the Federal Centers for Disease Control have been among youth 13 to 19 years of age (Centers for Disease Control 1988). However, given the lengthy latency period between infection and outbreak of classifiable symptoms of AIDS, a heavy proportion of 20- to 29-year-olds with AIDS (one-fifth of all reported AIDS cases) are presumed to have been infected with HIV as teenagers. Although adolescents are widely assumed to be a population at high risk for HIV infection and AIDS, direct data supporting this assumption are currently sparse. Accepted facts are these: 50 percent of high school men and 33 percent of high school women have engaged in sexual intercourse at least once (Hassner 1987). Condom use among adolescents for contraceptive purposes is known to be sporadic, with less than one-third of adolescents reporting contraception use at last intercourse (Hofferth and Hayes 1987), and over a quarter in some studies reporting never using contraceptives at all (Planned Parenthood 1986). Adolescents' use of condoms for prophylactic (as opposed to contraceptive) purposes is not documented, but rates of prophylactic use are widely assumed to be low. Incidence rates for anal intercourse and other high-risk sexual activities among teenagers have not been established.

With regard to drug-related risk factors, even the relatively more complete information available on adolescent drug use does not as yet shed clear light on incidence of intravenous drug use, needle sharing, or the culture of such activities among school-age youth. Recent survey data show that 57 percent of high school seniors in 1986 reported using illicit drugs at least once and that about one-third had used illicit drugs other than marijuana (Bachman et al. 1987). This is the highest illicit drug use rate among adolescents in any industrialized country (Johnston, personal communication). Such data are particularly disquieting given the fact that a large proportion of the highest-drug-using adolescents drop out of school prior to their senior year and thus are not counted in this survey report.

The plethora of drug-use questionnaires administered to school-age youth in recent years most commonly ask about ever-use and frequency of use of certain substances, but only rarely probe for data on adolescents' preferred methods for drug administration. Commonly, such drugs as cocaine are available in forms to be snorted, smoked, injected, or topically applied. Thus, data simply on frequency of use of cocaine or use at any time in the last month do not contribute a great deal to establishing frequency of needle use in various adolescent subgroups. Further, a variety of studies outline the disinhibiting effects of many substances on sexual behavior (Howard 1982; Room and Collins 1983; Stall et al. 1986). Thus, even non-IV drug use may play a significant role in precipitating or maintaining an adolescent's exposure to HIV. Issues related to the interaction of drug use and high-risk sexual behavior among adolescents are underresearched and currently not of much assistance to program planners or prevention researchers.

A few recent studies report knowledge levels and understanding of HIV and AIDS among students in middle and senior high schools. Data collected in 1984 revealed mass media as the primary source of

151

AIDS information for a high school sample of 250 (Price et al. 1985). Students in this study were both uninformed and misinformed about the disease. The researchers concluded that provision of accurate and complete information in the public schools was a desirable and necessary corrective to frequently superficial coverage of AIDS in the mass media that led to student misperceptions.

A 1986 study from San Francisco (n=1,326) showed that, even in an urban setting where AIDS has had high and long-standing visibility, there was marked variability in high school students' knowledge of AIDS and in their understanding of the precautionary measures that may reduce risk of HIV infection (DiClemente et al. 1986). The study's authors emphasize the need to overcome students' misperceptions by öffering school-based instruction on AIDS as part of a comprehensive teaching plan to instruct students about communicable diseases in general and the role of social values in controlling sexually transmitted diseases in particular. A second study of San Francisco high school students (n=628) found substantial ethnic differences in students' knowledge of AIDS (DiClemente et al. 1988). The research team concluded that black and Latino students were approximately twice as likely as white students to have misconceptions about the casual transmission of AIDS and that black and Latino youth may be at greater risk of HIV infection as a consequence of engaging in unsafe sexual practices attributable to insufficient information.

To date, few if any studies have linked knowledge and attitudes about AIDS with adolescents' reports of their own sexual and drug-using behavior. No evaluations of drug prevention programs for adolescents containing an AIDS component could be located for this report.

FACTORS COMPLICATING EFFECTIVE AIDS PREVENTION IN SCHOOLS

Second only to families, schools are the primary socializing influence for children and adolescents in our society. Schools allow ready access to the majority of this Nation's adolescents through huge, well-established educational service delivery systems. Schools are well-respected local institutions, touching all families in a community regardless of race, ethnicity, or income. There is some evidence that programs initiated in school settings can reach through students to engage and alter the health behavior of whole families (Nader et al. 1982; Perry 1986). Through schools, it is possible to present sequenced curriculum over a span of several years to reinforce and expand learning in developmentally appropriate ways. Finally, schools provide the best system for screening, early detection, and remedial or ameliorative assistance to children and youth with high potential for future health and behavior problems (Kirschenbaum 1983). For these reasons, schools are almost universally seen as principal sites for primary prevention of a wide variety of social and health problems, including AIDS.

Nonetheless, several realities have limited the effectiveness of school-based prevention programs. Adolescents at highest risk for most problem behaviors are those who are most alienated from this community institution. For example, youth most at risk for AIDS through drug use—early substance users; children and partners of substance users; black, Latino, and Native American youth; delinquent youth; and runaways—are most apt to drop out of school or attend school too sporadically to be reached by typical classroom-based prevention programs (Pirie et al. 1988; Zabin et al. 1986). Further, as community institutions, schools and school programs can become battlefields involving parents and community groups who, on moral or religious grounds, object to instructional programs for youth that contain information on sex, contraception, homosexuality, and drugs (Gilchrist and Schinke 1983b; Lamers 1988). To be effective in reducing the spread of AIDS, educational materials and programs must be clear and explicit. But the mechanisms of AIDS transmission raise moral, religious, and sexual issues that are uncomfortable or outright threatening for many adults (Lamers 1988) and the explicitness of some AIDS educational materials have been criticized by some community groups.

Thus, even when mandated by the U.S. Surgeon General, school-based programs on sensitive and value-laden issues can be difficult to design and launch. Teachers themselves resist involvement in such programs on the grounds that they are unprepared to address new politically loaded and complex psychosocial and behavioral topics (Smith et al. 1984). The complexity of school systems and school administrative structures in themselves limit the capacity of schools to make rapid change. Thus, incorporation of new programs is a slow process. Finally, economic factors play a part in constricting traditional school-based primary and secondary prevention programs. Time constraints and funding limitations result in the fact that health education programs, including sex education, life skills courses, and early intervention, are the first to be cut in favor of preserving basic instruction in the three R's. Even when specially funded research and demonstration programs produce positive results and enthusiastic local support, such programs are routinely discontinued when the special or supplementary funding ends.

DOCUMENTED SCHOOL-BASED PREVENTION PROGRAMS FOR ADOLESCENTS

School-based prevention programs reported in the extensive literature on health promotion and disease or problem prevention can be grouped into two categories: self-contained programs offered to adolescents by and in the schools that extend only minimally outside the school, and school programs that are but one facet of a comprehensive, integrated, multicomponent, communitywide prevention effort.

School-Only Programs

The most sophisticated school-only prevention programs to date involve smoking prevention. These programs typically involve one of two related approaches: social inoculation (Flay 1985a; Flay 1985b) and social skills development (Botvin and Wills 1985; Schinke et al. 1985). The inoculation approach involves anticipating and learning to refute social pressure and to manage difficult life situations in advance of encountering them. The skills-building approaches emphasize enhancing positive interpersonal interactions to increase adolescents' self-esteem and sense of self-efficacy. Descriptions of the social inoculation and social skills development approaches are available in other NIDA monographs (Bell and Battjes 1985; Glynn et al. 1983) and will not be reviewed here. Evaluations of variations on these two approaches demonstrate positive preventive effects for up to 3 years postintervention. These smoking prevention studies have been large and complex. Several thoughtful analyses of methodological weaknesses in the research on these programs mitigate but do not reduce confidence in their positive findings and provide detailed plans for improving methodology in future school-based ventures (Biglan and Ary 1985; Biglan et al. 1987; Flay 1985b; McCaul and Glasgow 1985).

Reports of findings and experiences with school-only programs that focus on drugs other than smoking have had less clear results (Goodstadt 1986; Moskowitz 1983; Schaps et al. 1981; Tobler 1986; Williams et al. 1985). Tobler's (1986) meta-analysis covering 147 studies provides a useful review of almost two decades of research on drug prevention research. Her quantitative analysis concludes that, for the average school-based adolescent population, programs with a peer-leader focus achieved and maintained the largest positive effects on participants' use of cigarettes, alcohol, and soft and hard drugs.

154

On the other hand, for at-risk adolescents (juvenile delinquents, drug abusers, and students with school problems), the most effective programs were those that went beyond what school settings usually provide to give adolescents experience with individualized alternatives to drug use—e.g., job and academic skills training, physical activities to increase students' sense of competence and control over their environments.

A recent qualitative analysis of school-only drug education programs notes a general lack of lasting, positive program effects (Goodstadt 1986). The author points to failures to appreciate, at the program planning stage, that students represent a range of motivation and experience with respect to drug use. Prevention programs proceed as though classes were comprised exclusively of nonusers, and program evaluations have failed to examine possible differences in the short- and long-term response of separate student subgroups. Goodstadt (1986) and others (Biglan and Ary 1985; Gullotta and Adams 1982) take prevention program developers to task for failing to make the necessary links between the reality of the classroom and the reality outside the classroom. These same authors criticize the failure to take into account the wide array of individual differences in subjects' beliefs, abilities, aspirations, intentions, and perception of social norms. These failures sharply reduce many programs' long-term effectiveness in reducing drug use and abuse.

Most school programs have focused on increasing adolescents' information base, interpersonal skills, and motivation to avoid drugs and other forms of behavior that place them at risk. The majority of drug prevention programs address the so-called gateway drugs: cigarettes, alcohol, and marijuana. The rationale used by these programs is that helping adolescents avoid the first steps in the typical progression from licit to illicit drug use will reduce the number of students who eventually move to regular and habitual hard drug use, including intravenous drug administration.

Although the vast majority of school sex-education programs have not been formally evaluated, two school-based approaches focused on decreasing adolescents' risk in the area of sexual behavior have had positive results. One approach involves skills building. A series of studies testing a cognitive/behavioral skills building program to increase adolescents' refusal of sexual intercourse and to increase their negotiation and use of effective contraception during intercourse demonstrated that adolescents can be taught to engage in protected sex practices (Gilchrist and Schinke 1983a; Gilchrist et al. 1987; Schinke et al. 1981). This cognitive/behavioral skills building approach is currently receiving further testing in 20 California school districts. The other approach is what might be called environmental modification. A survey of over 35 school-based programs in several geographic areas showed that, when certain confidentiality measures were observed, more sexually active adolescents requested and effectively used contraception. The contraceptives dispensed by a health service site on school grounds were more effective when compared with request and compliance rates at health service centers located off school campuses (Kirby 1986).

School Programs Within Larger Communitywide Efforts

Decidedly fewer evaluations are available for prevention programs that make use of schools as one facet of a larger community-based approach. In a special issue of the *Journal of School Health* (November 1986), several researchers articulate excellent rationales for addressing multiple community institutions at one time to increase health and reduce problem behavior among adolescents (Perry 1986; Johnson 1986; Murray 1986; Pentz 1986; Orlandi 1986; Flay 1986; Griffin 1986). Common to the nascent community-based prevention approaches described is the analysis of social substructures that constitute and affect given communities. Also important is the planning of programs most appropriate for each substructure or community unit so that a collection of multipronged, specially tailored programs are launched simultaneously to reinforce, augment, and sustain one another (Flay 1986; Griffin 1986; Johnson 1986; Orlandi 1986; Pentz 1986; Perry 1986). Such community analysis for the purpose of designing specific marketing and intervention efforts to reach specific community segments grows out of work initiated at Stanford to devise broad-based methods for reducing risk factors for cardiovascular disease (Solomon and Maccoby 1984). Research evaluating such community-based health promotion programs is now ongoing in Minnesota (Blackburn et al. 1984; Murray 1986), Kansas (Pentz et al. 1986), Rhode Island (Lasater et al. 1984), California (Farquhar et al. 1984), and elsewhere.

Several studies on the etiology and treatment of opiate use stress the need to incorporate social and cultural knowledge about the lives of groups to whom drug prevention and treatment programs are addressed (Dembo and Shern 1982; Gersick et al. 1981; Kaufman 1978). Such knowledge seems particularly critical when addressing black and Latino inner-city adolescents who are at high risk both for adopting drug-involved lifestyles, for HIV transmission, and for AIDS. In a

156

series of studies, Dembo and his associates demonstrated the power of sociocultural and environmental factors, as opposed to disturbed-personality factors, as influences on the drug involvement of lower class, inner-city youth (Dembo et al. 1979; Dembo et al. 1978; Dembo et al. 1981; Dembo and Shern 1982). Unfortunately, most of the well-evaluated, community-based prevention programs to date have primarily focused on suburban, middle- or working-class communities. Few community-based prevention studies involving high-risk, low-income, inner-city groups have yet emerged.

One potential exception is an ongoing series of drug prevention studies with low-achieving, inner-city elementary school-age children. These studies focus on reducing a number of precursors or early risk factors known to be associated with drug experimentation and drug use in adolescence. Hawkins, Catalano, and associates are studying methods to ultimately reduce drug use by changing the social context in which at-risk children develop. This prevention strategy aims at low-achieving children in elementary schools. The strategy includes a component to teach teachers to alter classroom climate with reward and punishment structures. In addition, a component has been developed to help students' parents increase their monitoring and communication skills, develop appropriate expectations for their child, and use fair and consistent discipline. This integrated school/home prevention program is designed to decrease family conflict and school failure and increase students' bonding to prosocial (i.e., antidrug) institutions and influences, namely schools and family. Although still being evaluated, this approach and emphasis on modifying social context and social bonding has produced initial positive effects (Hawkins and Catalano 1987; Hawkins et al., in press).

ANECDOTAL EXPERIENCES RELATED TO AIDS AND HIV TRANSMISSION

Because alterations in formal school curricula take time to initiate and implement, those schools that address AIDS education typically do so with single-shot programs for seniors or, in some cases, for an entire high school student body. Unpublished data from Washington State show that high school students' knowledge can be reliably increased with as little as 1 hour of instruction specifically about AIDS and HIV transmission (Miller and Downer, in press). Occasionally, one-shot school programs incorporate a mailing to students' homes containing information about AIDS and HIV transmission with encouragement to parents to discuss AIDS with their children. The effects of such mailed encouragements are not well-documented.

Despite this gap in data, the drawbacks of the one-shot health education approach are well known. First, one-shot programs must be exceptionally well done to hold student attention. For developmental reasons, a great many students do not see themselves at risk for AIDS. Sexual identity and sexual functioning are not well established until late adolescence and early adulthood. For younger adolescents, feelings and fears surrounding sexual behavior are strong. Homosexuality is a singularly uncomfortable topic for adolescent males. Adolescents' difficulties in acknowledging and planning ahead for their own sexual behavior have long been recognized as a factor contributing to unintended pregnancies (Schinke et al. 1979). For both sexes, heterosexual encounters are most comfortable when they are "spontaneous" and unplanned (Gilchrist and Schinke 1983b). With regard to drugs, active intravenous needle use among adolescents who attend school regularly is relatively rare, and few youth in school intend to inject drugs. Thus, messages about anal intercourse, condom use, and needle sharing, when not rejected outright, seem remote and irrelevant to many students. Second, even when students attend to and learn from AIDS education programs, there may be no application of that knowledge to behavior and no reduction of risk for HIV transmission. For all age groups, changes in knowledge alone have not been reliably associated with protective behavior change (Kelly et al. 1987).

RECOMMENDED INTERVENTION MODELS

Intervention models must be appropriate to the goals that they are supposed to achieve. Available data (Flay 1985a) suggest that programs with a social/psychological framework, including both the social inoculation and social skills-building variations, can positively affect the behavior of many mainstream, middle-class school students. These interventions reduce students' risk of problems associated with substance use and, less certainly, with sexual behavior. To date, few if any findings suggest the presence of any unintended negative effects from these programs that would contraindicate widescale use. Nonetheless, the primary complaint about programs based on this model is that they fail to reach or to change the behavior of precisely those students at highest risk—early experimenters with sex and drugs, and students with school attendance problems. In-school interventions based on the social/psychological intervention paradigm thus may be useful for some but clearly not for all adolescents. Such school-based programs must be supplemented with other kinds of risk reduction programs aimed at youth not accessible through the school system.

A useful framework for extending thinking about a multipronged approach to AIDS risk reduction for adolescents may be found in scholarly work that considers program design on the basis of participants' risk potential and the probable cost effectiveness of program components (Gordon 1983; Schinke et al. 1986). This work outlines three types or measures of prevention/intervention programming.

> The most generally applicable type, which we shall call underline, is [an intervention] measure that is desirable for everybody. In this category fall all those measures which can be advocated confidently for the general public ... There are many measures, however, in which the balance of benefits against risk and cost is such that the procedure can be recommended only when the individual is a member of a subgroup ... whose risk of becoming ill is above average. These measures we shall call selective ... The third class of preventive measures, which we propose to term indicated, encompasses those that are advisable only for persons who, on examination, are found to manifest a risk factor. (Gordon 1983, p. 108.)

Within this intervention nosology, three types of AIDS- related intervention programs for adolescents appear useful to develop. First is the universal strategy or approach, using school classrooms in all schools to disseminate to all students: accurate information about HIV transmission and AIDS; information about anticipating situations containing risk; information about decisionmaking regarding personal behavior in those situations; and some practice with the skills necessary to implement safe decisions. This universal approach is broadest in scope, least intensive and costly, but also least likely to yield enduring behavior change. Such universal programs, however, may be sufficient for adolescents at reasonably low risk for infection.

A selective intervention strategy is recommended for reaching students whose risk for AIDS is above average. This strategy dictates special efforts in particular school districts (or in particular schools within one district) where drug use, delinquency, and pregnancy or sexually transmitted disease rates are higher than national averages. Adolescents in these schools may be assumed to be at greater than average risk and to require more than information and minimal skills building. Programs in these schools should incorporate more intensive programming, involving peer-led stress-management techniques, self-esteem building and communication skills development. Worth investigation is the incorporation of selective in-school intervention efforts as part of a coordinated risk reduction strategy that addresses all segments of a neighborhood or high-risk geographic community.

Third, special high intensity programs are needed for indicated popu-lations who are already engaging in behavior associated with HIV transmission. Schools are only peripherally useful sites for such pro-grams, which must address the needs of drug-using and sexually active dropouts, truants, runaways, young addicts, and other adoles-cents alienated—probably permanently—from schools. Social service agencies, detention centers, street shelters, support groups for gay and lesbian youth, community health centers, and mental health treat-ment facilities provide more useful access than schools to these high-est risk groups. Interventions with these adolescents will probably need to be highly personalized and supportive over long periods of time to affect and maintain behavior change that leads to consistent safety from HIV exposure and transmission.

Complicating all school program planning is the indisputable fact that student bodies are not homogeneous. Within the same school, differ-ent students are at differing levels of risk and thus require different kinds of intervention strategies. A single school, for example, may launch a low-intensity universal AIDS intervention program for all students and, concomitantly, a more intensive selective program for students enrolled in contract studies or other dropout prevention classes.

RECOMMENDED RESEARCH INITIATIVES

Epidemiological and ethnographic studies of risk behavior among a wide variety of adolescent subgroups are needed to determine adoles-cents' vulnerability to HIV transmission and to form the basis for selecting appropriate levels of school-based intervention. Available studies suggest, but do not definitively show, that a single interven-tion program can successfully reduce multiple risk behaviors among adolescents (Botvin 1983). Research might profitably focus on testing interventions that simultaneously address related risks, for example, drug use, sexual activity, unintended pregnancy, and sexually trans-mitted diseases. At the present time, most in-school interventions address only one risk factor at a time, resulting in fragmentation and too many competing liens on time within the instructional day.

Research might also profitably move from almost exclusive focus on intervention content to research on larger organizational and policy climate issues that support or impede preventive interventions

160

undertaken by schools. Such an expanded focus would include research on how schools can serve as foci, triggers, or complementary components in a coordinated communitywide AIDS awareness and prevention effort.

REFERENCES

Bachman, J.G.; Johnston, L. D.; and O'Malley, P.M. *Monitoring the Future: Questionnaire Responses from the Nation's High School Seniors: 1986.* Ann Arbor: University of Michigan, Institute for Social Research, 1987. 279 pp.

Bell, C.S., and Battjes, R., eds. *Prevention Research: Deterring Drug Abuse Among Children and Adolescents.* National Institute on Drug Abuse Research Monograph 63. DHHS Pub. No. (ADM)85-1334. Washington, DC: Supt. of Docs., U.S. Govt. Print. Off., 1985. 235 pp.

Biglan, A., and Ary, D.V. Methodological issues in research on smoking prevention. In: Bell, C.S., and Battjes, R., eds. *Prevention Research: Deterring Drug Abuse Among Children and Adolescents.* National Institute on Drug Abuse Research Monograph 63. DHHS Pub. No. (ADM)85-1334. Washington, DC: Supt. of Docs., U.S. Govt. Print. Off., 1985. pp. 170-195.

Biglan, A.; Severson, H.; Ary, D.; Faller, C.; Gallison, C.; Thompson, R.; Glasgow, R.; and Lichtenstein, E. Do smoking prevention programs really work? Attrition and the internal and external validity of an evaluation of a refusal skills training program. *J Behav Med* 10:159-171, 1987.

Blackburn, H.; Luepker, R.V.; Kline, F.G.; Bracht, N.; Carlaw, R.; Jacobs, D.; Mittelmark, M.; Stauffer, L.; and Taylor, H.L. The Minnesota Heart Health Program: A research and demonstration project in cardiovascular disease prevention. In: Matarazzo, J.D.; Weiss, Steven M.; Herd, J.A.; Miller, N.E.; and Weiss, Sharlene M., eds. *Behavioral Health: A Handbook of Health Enhancement and Disease Prevention.* New York: John Wiley, 1984. pp. 1171-1178.

Botvin, G.J. Prevention of adolescent substance abuse through the development of personal and social competence. In: Glynn, T.J.; Leukefeld, C.G.; and Ludford, J.P., eds. *Preventing Adolescent Drug Abuse: Intervention Strategies.* National Institute on Drug Abuse Research Monograph 47. DHEW Pub. No. (ADM) 83-1280. Washington, DC: Supt. of Docs., U.S. Govt. Print. Off., 1983. pp. 115-140.

Botvin, G.J., and Wills, T.A. Personal and social skills training: Cognitive-behavioral approaches to substance abuse prevention. In: Bell, C.S., and Battjes, R., eds. *Prevention Research: Deterring Drug Abuse Among Children and Adolescents.* National Institute on Drug Abuse Research Monograph 63. DHHS Pub. No. (ADM)85-1334. Washington, DC: Supt. of Docs., U.S. Govt. Print. Off., 1985. pp. 8-49.

Centers for Disease Control. *AIDS Weekly Surveillance Report.* U.S. AIDS Program, Center for Infectious Diseases, March 21, 1988. p. 5.

Dembo, R.; Farrow, D.; Des Jarlais, D.; Burgos, W.; and Schmeidler, J. Examining a causal model of early drug involvement among inner city junior high school youths. *Human Relations* 34:169-193, 1981.

Dembo, R.; Farrow, D.; Schmeidler, J.; and Burgos, W. 1979. Testing a causal model of environmental influences on the early drug involvement of inner city junior high school youths. *Am J Drug Alcohol Abuse* 6:313-336, 1979.

Dembo, R.; Schmeidler, J.; and Burgos, W. Factors in the drug involvement of inner city junior high school youths: A discriminant analysis. Presented at the Fifth National Drug Abuse Conference, Seattle, WA, April 1978.

Dembo, R., and Shern, D. Relative deviance and the process(es) of drug involvement among inner-city youths. *Int J Addict* 17:1373-1399, 1982.

DiClemente, R.J.; Boyer, C.B.; and Morales, E.S. Minorities and AIDS: Knowledge, attitudes, and misconceptions among Black and Latino adolescents. *Am J Public Health* 78:55-57, 1988.

DiClemente, R.J.; Zorn, J.; and Temoshok, L. Adolescents and AIDS: A survey of knowledge, attitudes and beliefs about AIDS in San Francisco. *Am J Public Health* 76:1443-1445, 1986.

Farquhar, J.W.; Fortmann, S.P.; Maccoby, N.; et al. The Stanford Five City Project: An overview. In: Matarazzo, J.D.; Weiss, Steven M.; Herd, J.A.; Miller, N.E.; and Weiss, Sharlene M., eds. *Behavioral Health: A Handbook of Health Enhancement and Disease Prevention.* New York: John Wiley, 1984. pp. 1154-1165.

Flay, B.R. Psychosocial approaches to smoking prevention: A review of findings. *Health Psychol* 4:449-488, 1985a.

Flay, B.R. What we know about the social influences approach to smoking prevention: Review and recommendations. In: Bell, C.S., and Battjes, R., eds. *Prevention Research: Deterring Drug Abuse Among Children and Adolescents.* National Institute on Drug Abuse Research Monograph 63. DHHS Pub. No. (ADM)85-1334. Washington, DC: Supt. of Docs., U.S. Govt. Print. Off., 1985b. pp. 67-112.

Flay, B.R. Mass media linkages with school-based programs for drug abuse prevention. *J Sch Health* 56:402-406, 1986.

Gersick, K.E.; Grady, K.; Sexton, E.; and Lyons, M. Personality and sociodemographic factors in adolescent drug use. In: Lettieri, D.J., and Ludford, J.P., eds. *Drug Abuse and the American Adolescent.* National Institute on Drug Abuse Research Monograph 38. DHHS Pub. No. (ADM)81-1166. Washington, DC: Supt. of Docs., U.S. Govt. Print. Off., 1981. pp. 39-56.

Gilchrist, L.D., and Schinke, S.P. Coping with contraception: Cognitive and behavioral methods with adolescents. *Cognitive Ther Res* 7:379-388, 1983a.

Gilchrist, L.D., and Schinke, S.P. Teenage pregnancy and public policy. *Soc Serv Rev* 57:307-322, 1983b.

Gilchrist, L.D.; Schinke, S.P.; and Maxwell, J.S. Life skills counseling for preventing problems in adolescence. *J Soc Serv Res* 10(2-4):73-84, 1987.

Glynn, T.J.; Leukefeld, C.G.; and Ludford, J.P., eds. *Preventing Adolescent Drug Abuse: Intervention Strategies.* National Institute on Drug Abuse Research Monograph 47. DHEW Pub. No. (ADM) 83-1280. Washington, DC: Supt. of Docs., U.S. Govt. Print. Off., 1983. 261 pp.

Goodstadt, M.S. School-based drug education in North America: What is wrong? What can be done? *J Sch Health* 56:278-281, 1986.

Gordon, R.S., Jr. An operational classification of disease prevention. *Public Health Rep* 98:107-109, 1983.

Griffin, T. Community-based chemical use problem prevention. *J Sch Health* 56:414-417, 1986.

Gullotta, T., and Adams, G.R. Substance abuse minimization: Conceptualizing prevention in adolescent and youth programs. *J Youth Adolescence* 11:409-424, 1982.

Hassner, D.W. *AIDS and Adolescents: The Time for Prevention is Now.* Washington, DC: Center for Population Options, 1987. 261 pp.

Hawkins, J.D., and Catalano, R.F. The Seattle Social Development Project: Progress report on a longitudinal prevention study. Presented at the National Institute on Drug Abuse Science Press Seminar, Washington, DC, March 1987.

Hawkins, J.D.; Doueck, H.J.; and Lishner, D.M. Changing teaching practices in mainstream classrooms to improve bonding and behavior of low achievers. *American Educational Research Journal* 25(1):31-50, 1988.

Hofferth, S.L., and Hayes, C.D., eds. *Risking the Future: Adolescent Sexuality, Pregnancy, and Childbearing: Statistical Appendixes.* Washington, DC: National Academy Press, 1987. 168 pp.

Howard, M. *Did I Have a Good Time? Teenage Drinking.* New York: Continuum, 1982. 159 pp.

Iverson, D.C., and Kolbe, L.J. Evolution of the national disease prevention and health promotion strategy: Establishing a role for the schools. *J Sch Health* 53:294-302, 1983.

Johnson, C.A. Objectives of community programs to prevent drug abuse. *J Sch Health* 56:364-368, 1986.

Kaufman, E. The relationship of social class and ethnicity to drug abuse. In: Smith, D.E.; Anderson, S.M.; Buxton, M.; Gottlieb, N.; Harvey, W.; and Chung, T., eds. *A Multicultural View of Drug Abuse.* Cambridge, MA: Shenkman, 1978. 362 pp.

Kelly, J.A.; St. Lawrence, J.S.; Brafield, T.L.; and Hood, M.V. Relationships between knowledge about AIDS risk and actual behavior in a sample of homosexual men: Implications for prevention. Presented at the 3rd International Conference on AIDS, Washington, DC, June 1987.

Kirby, D. Comprehensive school-based health clinics: A growing movement to improve adolescent health and reduce teen-age pregnancy. *J Sch Health* 56:289-291, 1986.

Kirschenbaum, D.S. Toward more behavioral early intervention programs: A rationale. *Professional Psychol: Res Practice* 14:159-169, 1983.

Lamers, E.P. Public schools confront AIDS. In: Corless, I.B., and Pittman-Lindeman, M., eds. *AIDS: Principles, Practices, and Politics.* Washington, DC: Hemisphere, 1988. pp. 175-185.

Lasater, T.; Abrams, D.; Artz, L.; et al. Lay volunteer delivery of a community-based cardiovascular risk factor change program: The Pawtucket Experiment. In: Matarazzo, J.D.; Weiss, Steven M.; Herd, J.A.; Miller, N.E.; and Weiss, Sharlene M., eds. *Behavioral Health: A Handbook of Health Enhancement and Disease Prevention.* New York: John Wiley, 1984. pp. 1166-1170.

McCaul, K.D., and Glasgow, R.E. Preventing adolescent smoking: What have we learned about treatment construct validity? *Health Psychol* 4:361-387, 1985.

Miller, L., and Downer, A. Knowledge and attitude changes in adolescents following one hour of AIDS instruction. Seattle, WA: Seattle-King County Department of Public Health, AIDS Prevention Project. Unpublished manuscript.

Moskowitz, J.M. Preventing adolescent substance abuse through drug education. In: Glynn, T.J.; Leukefeld, C.G.; and Ludford, J.P., eds. *Preventing Adolescent Drug Abuse: Intervention Strategies.* National Institute on Drug Abuse Research Monograph 47. DHEW Pub. No. (ADM)83-1280. Washington, DC: Supt. of Docs., U.S. Govt. Print. Off., 1983. pp. 233-249.

Murray, D.M. Dissemination of community health promotion programs: The Fargo-Moorhead Heart Health Program. *J Sch Health* 56:375-381, 1986.

Nader, P.R.; Perry, C.; Maccoby, N.; Solomon, D.; Killen, J.; Telch, M.; and Alexander, J.K. Adolescent perceptions of family health behavior: A tenth grade educational activity to increase family awareness of a community cardiovascular risk reduction program. *J Sch Health* 52:372-377, 1982.

Orlandi, M.A. Community-based substance abuse prevention: A multicultural perspective. *J Sch Health* 56:394-401, 1986.

Pentz, M.A. Community organization and school liaisons: How to get programs started. *J Sch Health* 56:382-388, 1986.

Pentz, M.A.; Cormack, C.; Flay, B.; Hansen, W.B.; and Johnson, C.A. Balancing program and research integrity in community drug abuse prevention: Project STAR approach. *J Sch Health* 56:389-393, 1986.

Perry, C.L. Community-wide health promotion and drug abuse prevention. *J Sch Health* 56:359-363, 1986.

Pirie, P.L.; Murray, D.M.; and Luepker, R.V. Smoking prevalence in a cohort of adolescents, including absentees, dropouts, and transfers. *Am J Public Health* 78:176-178, 1988.

Planned Parenthood. *American Teens Speak: Sex, Myths, TV, and Birth Control.* Planned Parenthood Federation of America, Inc., 1986. 86 pp.

Price, J.H.; Desmond, S.; and Kukulka, G. High school students' perceptions and misperceptions of AIDS. *J Sch Health* 55:107-109, 1985.

Room, R., and Collins, G. *Alcohol and Disinhibition: Nature and Meaning of the Link.* National Institute on Alcoholism and Alcohol Abuse Research Monograph 12. DHEW Pub. No. (ADM)83-1246. Washington, DC: Supt. of Docs., U.S. Govt. Print. Off., 1983. 505 pp.

Schaps, E.; DiBartolo, R.; Moskowitz, J.; et al. A review of 127 drug abuse prevention program evaluations. *J Drug Issues* 11:17-43, 1981.

Schinke, S.P.; Blythe, B.J.; and Gilchrist, L.D. Cognitive-behavioral prevention of adolescent pregnancy. *Journal of Counseling Psychology* 28:451-454, 1981.

Schinke, S.P.; Gilchrist, L.D.; and Small, R.W. Preventing unwanted adolescent pregnancy: A cognitive-behavioral approach. *Amer J Orthopsychiatry* 49:81-88, 1979.

Schinke, S.P.; Gilchrist, L.D.; and Snow, W.H. Skills intervention to prevent cigarette smoking among adolescents. *Am J Public Health* 75:665-667, 1985.

Schinke, S.P.; Schilling, R.F., II; Gilchrist, L.D.; Whittaker, J.K.; Kirkham, M.A.; Senechal, V.A.; Snow, W.H.; and Maxwell, J.S. Definitions and methods for prevention research with youth and families. *Children and Youth Services Review* 8:257-266, 1986.

Smith, P.B.; Flaherty, C.; Webb, L.J.; and Mumford, D.M. The long-term effects of human sexuality training programs for public school teachers. *J Sch Health* 54:157-159, 1984.

Solomon, D.S., and Maccoby, N. Communication as a model for health enhancement. In: Matarazzo, J.D.; Weiss, Steven M.; Herd, J.A.; Miller, N.E.; and Weiss, Sharlene M., eds. *Behavioral Health: A Handbook of Health Enhancement and Disease Prevention.* New York: John Wiley, 1984. pp. 209-221.

Stall, R.; McKusick, L.; Wiley, J.; Coates, T.J.; and Ostrow, D.G. Alcohol and drug use during sexual activity and compliance with safe sex guidelines for AIDS: The AIDS behavioral research project. *Health Educ Q* 13:359-371, 1986.

Tobler, N.S. Meta-analysis of 143 adolescent drug prevention programs: Quantitative outcome results of program participants compared to a control or comparison group. *J Drug Issues* 16:537-567, 1986.

Williams, R.E.; Ward, D.A.; and Gray, L.N. The persistence of experimentally induced cognitive change: A neglected dimension in the assessment of drug prevention programs. *J Drug Educ* 15:33-42, 1985.

Zabin, L.S.; Hardy, J.B.; Smith, E.A.; and Hirsch, M.B. Substance use and its relation to sexual activity among inner-city adolescents. *J Adolesc Health Care* 7:320-331, 1986.

AUTHOR

Lewayne D. Gilchrist, Ph.D.
School of Social Work
University of Washington
4101 15th Avenue, N.E., JN-30
Seattle, WA 98195

The Role of Drug Abuse Treatment Programs in AIDS Prevention and Education Programs for Intravenous Drug Users: The New Jersey Experience

Joyce F. Jackson, Leslie G. Rotkiewicz, and Robert C. Baxter

INTRODUCTION

It is estimated that as many as 150,000 people in New Jersey may already have been infected with human immunodeficiency virus (HIV), the virus that causes acquired immunodeficiency syndrome (AIDS) (New Jersey State Department of Health 1987a). State Health Commissioner Molly Coye, in her "AIDS Toll Forecast," has indicated that approximately 1 in every 75 New Jerseyans may be infected (Star-Ledger 1987). Many of these exposed individuals unknowingly carry and transmit HIV to other persons. In New Jersey, HIV transmission is primarily through intravenous (IV) drug use or sexual intercourse among needle-sharing addicts. Unfortunately, symptoms of HIV exposure may not appear until 5 or more years after contamination. It is therefore possible for HIV carriers to show no signs or symptoms of AIDS for extended periods, but still transmit the virus (New Jersey State Department of Health 1987a). Based upon the present pattern of this disease, the total number of reported AIDS cases in New Jersey is likely to reach 20,000 by late 1991 (Star-Ledger 1987).

This perplexing viral phenomenon has contributed to the seemingly uncontrollable spread of HIV among primary risk groups, especially intravenous drug users (IVDUs). The dynamic infectious process, as well as sexual and drug abuse lifestyles, confound attempts to control the spread of AIDS in New Jersey. As with any infectious disease, understanding the complex interaction of "pathogen, host, and environment" is essential for developing solutions (Selwyn 1986).

In 1984, Weiss and colleagues (1986) conducted an HIV seroprevalence study among drug abuse patients enrolled in New Jersey treatment programs. This study revealed that 29 to 56 percent of the tested patients in the northeastern part of the State were HIV positive, with the HIV seropositivity percentage among New Jersey IVDUs in treatment decreasing as distance from New York City increases. Today, HIV infection rates are believed to be higher, although this has not been systematically determined. Preliminary results from a recent study of "small samples" of drug users from two major north- east cities in New Jersey indicate HIV seroprevalence of 47 percent and 60 percent (French 1988). According to the State Department of Health, approximately 76 percent of reported AIDS cases in New Jersey are found in the northeastern part of the State. This is the same area where the majority of IVDUs reside. Also, a recent study by the National Institute on Drug Abuse elsewhere in New Jersey found seroprevalence rates of 43 percent and 12 percent in two cities (Battjes, personal communication). The spread of the AIDS virus among IVDUs appears unabated, with the likelihood of transmission through shared needles and sexual contact increasing as more active abusers become infected (Weiss et al. 1986).

New Jersey currently ranks fifth in the Nation in total AIDS cases, with 3,462 cases reported as of January 31, 1988. Of those, approxi- mately 1,450 are still living and in need of various medical and com- munity support services. The composition of these cases in the State has been relatively stable since the beginning of the epidemic. As mentioned, New Jersey's AIDS population differs from national statis- tics in that the primary risk group is reported to be IVDUs. Indeed, Selwyn (1986) has indicated that approximately 80 percent of all IVDU AIDS-related cases in the Nation were reported from New York and New Jersey.

AIDS has already spread rapidly in New Jersey, with the number of reported cases increasing each year since 1981. During the past 5 months alone (July 1, 1987 to December 1, 1987), the rate increased 26 percent, with the reporting of 785 new cases (New Jersey State Department of Health 1987b). Although some of this is due to a change in the reporting definition by the Centers for Disease Control (CDC), effective September 1987, the rate of increase remains alarming.

Finally, the devastating consequences of AIDS infection among an increasing number of IVDUs is reflected in a growing number of pediatric AIDS cases. As of January 31, 1988, 91 percent of the

110 pediatric cases in New Jersey had a parent at risk for AIDS (New Jersey State Department of Health 1988), and New Jersey is second only to New York in total reported pediatric AIDS cases. The large majority of these cases are the result of maternal transmission from a mother who is an IVDU or a sexual partner of an abuser.

The preponderance of IVDU AIDS cases in New Jersey has resulted in a rather different demographic picture compared to the United States, generally. The following New Jersey statistics will serve to highlight these differences.

- Nineteen percent of our cases are among women, compared to only 7 percent nationally.

- Eight percent of cases are attributed to heterosexual transmission, compared to 4 percent nationally.

- Sixty-three percent of all cases are among blacks and Hispanics. Nationally, the percentage is 38.

- Ninety-one percent of children with AIDS are born to a parent with, or at risk for, AIDS. Nationally, this figure is also high at 76 percent.

- A little over 3 percent of our total cases are children with AIDS (under 13 years), compared to 1.5 percent nationally.

- Fifty-six percent of all reported AIDS cases are related to IV drug use as compared to approximately 25 percent nationally (New Jersey State Department of Health 1988).

Much has been learned about AIDS in recent years, but there is unfortunately no cure or anticipated vaccine to curtail this epidemic. Until a cure or vaccine is discovered, the only means of fighting this disease is to help individuals reduce their risk through mass media and specific prevention and education activities aimed at high-risk groups (New Jersey State Department of Health 1987a). It is hoped that increasing the AIDS knowledge level of the general public will result in a reduction in high-risk behavior. Those individuals who are in high-risk groups must also refrain from behavior that results in HIV transmission to others. AIDS information or education will serve no purpose unless it is translated into AIDS avoidance behavior.

Nationally, AIDS education and risk-reduction programs have already effected positive behavioral changes among various high-risk groups, including IVDUs (Selwyn 1986; Des Jarlais et al. 1988). However, much high-risk behavior continues among IVDUs. Unless methods to control the spread of HIV among IVDUs are established, many more will become ill and die, and this AIDS population will create a severe burden on the State's health care and social service systems.

Achieving lasting behavior change among IVDUs is a challenge. They tend to have more medical and social problems than other risk groups (Ginzburg 1988). Many IVDUs depend upon public assistance for financial and medical services. Often unemployed, they also frequently lack medical insurance and other benefits, housing, family support, and other financial reserves.

In other parts of our country, the predominant AIDS risk group is composed of homosexual men. The gay community has demonstrated an ability to organize voluntarily and provide resources and services to their cohorts across the Nation. IVDUs, on the other hand, generally lack the sophistication, literacy, group morale and resources, and political clout to mount comparable achievements in education, prevention, treatment, community support, and advocacy for their constituency (Jackson 1987). The inability of the drug-using community to organize and advocate for itself has forced the State Department of Health, nonprofit drug treatment programs, and other State agencies to provide AIDS-related services to IVDUs that are provided to the gay community by voluntary organizations.

Because the AIDS epidemic is associated with IV drug use and IVDUs' need for help in changing behavior, the New Jersey State Department of Health has developed treatment, prevention and education, and community support projects that are specifically aimed at special populations of IVDUs and their sexual partners. Efforts that utilize drug abuse treatment programs in AIDS prevention will be the focus of this paper.

HEROIN (IV) DRUG ABUSE SERVICES IN NEW JERSEY

The Division of Narcotic and Drug Abuse Control (DNDAC) of the State Department of Health has estimated that there were 40,000 IVDUs in New Jersey at any time from the seventies to the mid-eighties (New Jersey State Department of Health 1986), and this same estimate holds true in 1988. The cost to society of their addiction alone is estimated to be $750 million or more per year (New Jersey

State Department of Health 1985; Schadl, personal communication, 1988). There were 21,344 total drug abuse treatment admissions in 1980. Of those, 8,703 admissions were for outpatient heroin detoxification.

The Federal Government began reducing revenue designated for State drug abuse services in 1981. Because of this reduction, treatment services were decreased and a patient copayment obligation was introduced, resulting in a dramatic decline in heroin (IV) detoxification admissions. These economic and service barriers resulted in fewer minorities, especially black males, seeking drug abuse treatment (New Jersey State Department of Health 1986). Heroin detoxification admissions among black males declined 79 percent, from 3,643 in 1980 to only 777 in 1985. This is of particular concern, since minority groups are disproportionately represented in the number of AIDS cases in the State of New Jersey (New Jersey State Department of Health 1988). Since the seventies, it has been evident that numerous heroin addicts in New Jersey were willing to enter detoxification treatment if it were reasonably accessible.

AIDS Community Educator Program

The earliest outreach directed to the New Jersey IV drug-using community was begun in early 1985. This Community Health Education Project was established through a grant from the Federal CDC and involved the use of ex-addicts to reach active IVDUs in the streets. The goals of the Project were to disseminate information about AIDS to active IVDUs, stressing risk reduction with respect to sexual and childbearing behavior, and to develop a mechanism for feedback from active IVDUs to the drug treatment community on what is happening on the streets in regard to AIDS and drug abuse activities.

To carry out these project goals, contracts were generated with community-based drug treatment programs, including those that were drug-free residential, outpatient drug free, and methadone maintenance. By June 1985, eight former IVDUs (either drug free or methadone maintained) were hired on a half-time basis. These exaddict educators were chosen to function within geographic areas of New Jersey known to have varying numbers of AIDS cases and HIV seroprevalence ratio among IVDUs. There was a greater number of educators in northeastern New Jersey, where seroprevalence ratios in 1984 were known to be between 40 percent and 55 percent among IVDUs in drug treatment programs (Weiss et al. 1986). Other

171

educators were located in areas of low seroprevalence where it was considered important to conduct primarily preventive intervention.

Prior to beginning their field work, the ex-addict educators were trained in concepts such as the definition of AIDS, epidemiology and etiology of AIDS, modes of HIV transmission, the spectrum of HIV infection and related diseases, and risks reduction related to IV drug use and sexual behavior. Later, training was given in ethnography, and role playing was utilized to simulate situations that might occur on the streets.

After training, the community health educators were sent out into their communities to seek active street addicts and inform them about AIDS, how it is transmitted, and what they could do to decrease their chances of infection. The educators distributed literature on AIDS from the New Jersey State Department of Health and the U.S. Public Health Service, and acted as facilitators in bringing addicts into local drug treatment programs. The educators met monthly with the project coordinator to receive training, report on their work, and exchange information. Monthly reports detailing numbers of contacts, pieces of literature distributed, and observations were compiled by each community health educator.

Evaluation of the effect of the Project after the first 6 months came from direct reports from the ex-addict educators and from the results of a questionnaire administered to 577 IVDUs entering drug treatment programs to assess their level of knowledge about AIDS. The findings of the educators were as follows:

(1)   It is difficult to have an educational impact on IVDUs who are exhibiting compulsive drug-seeking behavior.

(2)   Large numbers of street addicts can be reached. Written materials had some importance because they could be read while users temporarily ceased their drug-seeking behavior.

(3)   For many addicts, enrollment in a treatment program is a prerequisite to achieve necessary behavior change on a regular basis.

(4)   More than half of addicts wanted treatment, but saw the cost as prohibitive.

The findings of the questionnaire (Ginzburg et al. 1986) administered between July and December 1985 were as follows:

(1)   White males and females tend to have better information about AIDS than either blacks or Hispanics.

(2)   Only 30 percent of respondents were aware that soaking needles and syringes in a bleach solution could reduce the risk of AIDS, but 82 percent knew that risk of infection could be reduced by not sharing "sets."

(3)   About half the respondents had correct knowledge of the major modes of transmission of AIDS. Blacks had the least awareness that AIDS can be spread by sexual relations.

(4)   Fifty-seven percent of the respondents were aware that babies born to IV users are at risk.

(5)   Fifteen percent of the respondents stated that a drug program field worker (ex-addict educator) was one of their sources of information on AIDS.

(6)   Almost half of the respondents were aware of major risk groups.

(7)   Poor knowledge of AIDS symptoms was demonstrated. More than 33 percent believed that those exposed to the AIDS virus would be visibly sick, and 66 percent believed that exposure would almost always result in death.

(8)   The most frequent responses for reasons for coming to treatment were "being tired of running" (68 percent) and "fear of AIDS and other diseases" (47 percent).

The Community Health Education Project has been expanded from the original 8 half-time educators to 28 full-time personnel. They are distributed throughout the State, but are concentrated in areas of high incidence of IV drug use and high HIV seropositivity (e.g., Essex and Hudson Counties). Over the past 2½ years, their roles and the messages they deliver have changed. Presently, they attempt to reach not only IVDUs, but also their sex partners. Although educators continue to warn of the dangers of needle sharing, the delivery of safer sex messages and warnings of the risk of infection to unborn children are stressed.

In many cases, the community health educators have become respected and valuable resources to the drug-using community. They assist
individuals in enrolling in drug treatment programs, help individuals
apply for entitlements, refer people to the HIV counseling and testing
sites, and advise symptomatic people about medical services available
at various clinics. Many educators are seen as the "AIDS person" by
the drug-using community and as a source of information and help to
this isolated population. Because they are hired directly by a
community-based program, they reflect the cultural and ethnic composition of the surrounding area. As discussed later, health educators
were invaluable in the implementation of New Jersey's coupon outreach program.

AIDS Coordinator Program

In 1985, the DNDAC began to develop the AIDS Coordinator Program
to address the growing problem of AIDS and the IVDU. The AIDS
Coordinator was used to provide professional expertise to coordinate
AIDS education and support services for IVDUs, drug program staffs,
patients, and community agencies with which they interface.

The 14 community-based drug treatment programs that already had
ex-addicts involved in the Community Health Education Project contracted with the Department of Health to hire individuals who had a
minimum of a bachelor's degree or were registered nurses. Prior to
beginning their work in March 1986, the AIDS Coordinators received
training that included medical aspects of AIDS, epidemiology and
modes of transmission, HIV antibody testing, social and psychological
issues, entitlements for patients with AIDS or AIDS-related complex
(ARC), and community networking techniques. Meetings and training
sessions were held monthly with program coordinators to discuss
their activities, attend workshops, and receive updates on AIDS
information.

The AIDS Coordinators' activities involved contact with substance
abusers in treatment, drug treatment program staff, and community
social service agencies, as well as the general community. They were
responsible for:

(1)   developing and implementing ongoing AIDS educational programs
        for patients and staff;

(2)   developing and implementing a program to identify, refer, and
        coordinate care of symptomatic patients;

(3)   assuring that supportive services such as family therapy and support groups were accessible and appropriate to drug abuse patients; and

(4)   networking with community agencies and serving as an educational resource.

The AIDS Coordinator Program was expanded from 14 to 28 full-time coordinators in January 1987. During November 1987 alone, coordinators conducted 948 educational sessions for clients, made 123 presentations in the community, conducted 588 individual AIDS counseling sessions, and made 307 AIDS-related referrals to medical and social services. Clearly, the AIDS Coordinator Program has become a vital and vocal force in New Jersey's multifaceted effort to confront the epidemic problem of AIDS and AIDS-related conditions among IVDUs, their sex partners, and their children.

One of the most important responsibilities of the AIDS Coordinator is the provision of AIDS education and risk reduction information to clients. The most obvious time to provide this education is at drug treatment admission, and many drug treatment programs in New Jersey have made AIDS education mandatory for new admissions. Although education at intake is essential, it should not be considered sufficient, nor is intake necessarily the most opportune time. Clients coming into treatment are often anxious; some may be feeling sick from drug withdrawal, and others may be preoccupied with the pressures that drove them into treatment in the first place (e.g., legal, family, or financial problems).

The AIDS Coordinator assures an ongoing program to support behavioral change. Many methadone programs, for example, have a phase system in which clients receive increased take-home privileges as they show progress in the program, and many residential drug-free programs "promote" clients based on their demonstration of responsible behavior. AIDS education is a mandatory requirement for advancement (promotion) in specific treatment programs.

Another significant time when AIDS education is appropriate is when observation or urinalysis indicates that clients are abusing drugs. Clients must be alerted to the dangers of continued drug use and warned that if they persist they may be discharged from the program. This discharge exposes them to increased AIDS risk. Indeed, this moment may be critical for AIDS education. Education is extremely important to the prevention of further HIV infection spread; however, education alone is often not sufficient to create and maintain behavioral change, particularly among IVDUs.

Drug treatment programs, therefore, need to develop systems to encourage and support behavioral change. Joint counseling sessions with clients and their sex partners and "safer sex" groups are methods that have been tried with varying degrees of success. Programs have been encouraged to try different approaches to determine what works for them. For example, one program tried separate safer sex groups for men and women and found separate groups were not well received. Few clients attended, and members' participation was limited. When the program began groups with men and women together, attendance grew, the groups became much more animated, and staff felt that the interactions were more positive and the pressure for behavioral change much stronger.

Coordinators have worked with a wide variety of formal and informal networks. Their efforts have resulted in the formation of community-based task forces in several communities—an important element in developing services and advocacy for a population that is without influential representation. Through the AIDS Coordinator Program, drug treatment agencies have widened their constituency and assumed a greater public health role in their communities.

The Coupon Program: Drug Treatment and AIDS Education

Based on statistics related to IV drug use, the transmission of AIDS, and the reduced percentage of minority males entering treatment since the imposition of client fees, the New Jersey State Department of Health determined that a program to entice heroin addicts into the treatment system was urgently needed. It was theorized that there were numerous heroin addicts in the inner city who would respond to free detoxification treatment. By eliminating the cost of treatment and assuring prompt service, a significant number of addicts who had been out of the treatment system for some time could be reached. Furthermore, it was anticipated that a number of these patients would continue in treatment beyond free detoxification. Finally, detoxification treatment that included an AIDS education component could provide opportunities to increase the AIDS knowledge level, change the behaviors of IVDUs, and thereby lower the probability of AIDS transmission among IVDUs and their sexual partners and/or needle-sharing partners.

A coupon program was developed to address that segment of the active drug abuse population either unable or unwilling to pay for heroin detoxification. This program involved the distribution of serially numbered detoxification coupons in areas where addiction was prevalent. Coupons valid for a specific program and time period were distributed through the previously established network of trained ex-addict community health educators.

Methadone programs received contracts to provide free heroin detoxification, up to 21 days, for all eligible heroin addicts who presented a valid coupon at intake. To be eligible, coupon bearers had to be addicted to the intravenous use of heroin and to have been without drug abuse treatment for the previous 12-month period. The program physician had final responsibility to determine eligibility, within State and Federal criteria.

Participating drug programs were required to provide 1 hour of AIDS education within the first 3 days of treatment to each person presenting a coupon. Additional program responsibilities included obtaining a brief sociodemographic history from each addict and administering pre- and post-AIDS education surveys to each coupon patient, to determine his or her understanding of the educational program's content. Posteducation surveys were conducted immediately after the AIDS education program.

Nine nonprofit methadone programs throughout the State participated in this pilot coupon project. The field project began in December 1986 and terminated March 31, 1987. Of the 1,000 detoxification coupons made available, 970 were distributed by the end of the program period. Of the distributed coupons, 84 percent were redeemed for heroin detoxification services. Thus, a total of 816 coupon questionnaires were evaluated.

Seventy-nine percent of the coupon recipients were males. The majority of the coupon program patients were black (66 percent), with white at 18 percent, and Hispanic at 16 percent. The mean age was 33.03 with a 6.4 standard deviation, and the age range was 18 to 63 years. Forty-five percent of the patients claimed no previous treatment attempts. The mean for the number of years since last treatment for those patients who claimed a previous treatment episode was 5.4 or mid-1981 with a 4.03 standard deviation (Jackson et al., in press).

177

Of the 816 patients who entered treatment via the coupon program, 95 percent received 1 hour of AIDS education. When pre- and post-AIDS education surveys were compared, significant improvement was shown in understanding on almost all AIDS knowledge questions. Ninety-five percent were initially aware of their IVDU risk-group status, but were considerably less aware of AIDS transmission to babies of IVDUs, female sex partners, and male sex partners. Coupon patients showed marked improvement in recognizing symptoms of AIDS. Blacks and Hispanics showed lower initial understanding of AIDS, but all improved at posttesting.

Data were also gathered at each participating program site to identify those coupon program participants who, as of May 1987, had continued in treatment beyond their coupon detoxification attempt. "Continuation in treatment" was defined as either acceptance into a methadone maintenance program or an additional detoxification attempt. Since the numbers of patients in all programs exceeded their funded capacity, little effort was made to retain patients beyond the detoxification period. Yet, 28 percent of the coupon recipients continued in treatment (Jackson et al., in press).

Subsequently, additional coupons were distributed. The coupon program was expanded from 9 original programs to 16 participating programs throughout the State. During 1987, approximately 2,000 IVDUs benefited from the coupon program. State AIDS prevention and education funding was used to support this project, which is expected to continue on an annual basis.

Mobile Health Vans

It is difficult for many residents of the inner city to reach health services and receive health education. This is especially true for IVDUs. In many cases, hospital emergency rooms are the primary providers of health care and information to the indigent. Emergency room interactions are often brief and, in the case of addicts, marked by mutual antipathy.

The Mobile Van Program of the New Jersey State Department of Health is designed to ameliorate this situation by providing education, information, and referral services for a broad range of health concerns to residents of inner-city neighborhoods. This outreach effort is aimed at drug users, their sexual partners, and significant others, to provide education, prevention, and early intervention services with respect to AIDS and substance abuse. Literature about and referral

178

to other health and social welfare concerns are also available from the van.

Two community-based drug treatment programs, one a methadone program and the other a therapeutic community, both located in areas of high seroprevalence for HIV infection and high incidence of IV drug use (Newark and Jersey City), received State monies for mobile van units. Funds were provided to purchase, equip, insure, and staff each van for approximately 3 days of operation a week.

Each van is staffed at all times by a driver, a trained counselor, and a physician. Upper-body physical examinations are conducted when indicated, and medical information and referrals provided when appropriate. No drugs are carried on the vans and no prescriptions are written by the mobile unit physicians. Each van is equipped with a two-way communication system between van and clinic so that the system is aware of the van's location. These services are provided on an anonymous basis; no identifying information or names are solicited. Serially numbered contact forms are completed for each person utilizing the van to facilitate the collection of statistical information and the evaluation of the project.

The van services are publicized through the media and by outreach to community agencies, tenants' associations, and church groups. In addition, the community health educators distribute flyers to drug users and their associates.

The first van became fully operational in August of 1987 and the second in December of 1987. Thus far, the vans have visited 44 different sites and served over 600 clients. Analysis of the contact sheets collected in December from both vans indicates that 74 percent of those using the vans' services were black, 15 percent were Hispanic, and 12 percent were white. Clients were almost equally divided between male and female (52 percent male and 48 percent female). Significantly, only 11 percent of the clients had any previous exposure to AIDS information or services, despite the fact that 40 percent of them said they themselves had engaged in high-risk behaviors (26 percent through IV drug use; 74 percent as sex partners of IVDUs). Almost a third had either a friend or a relative who was at risk.

Analysis of the data collected by mobile van units will be undertaken in the future; however, preliminary data indicate that vans are reaching persons at high risk for HIV infection either through IV drug use or as sex partners of IVDUs; they are being reached because service comes to them in their neighborhood. Almost 50 percent of those utilizing the vans' services did so because they saw it on the street, rather than just having been told about it or through publicity. The vans have been well received by the communities and community organizations, and tenant groups are requesting that vans visit their neighborhoods.

SPECIAL SERVICES FOR IVDUS WITH AIDS AND ARC

In addition to the AIDS prevention initiatives described above, drug abuse treatment programs in New Jersey are beginning to provide special services for IVDUs who have AIDS or ARC.

Residential Beds

Because there are proportionately more indigent and homeless people among IVDUs than among any other AIDS risk group, the burden on New Jersey hospitals treating AIDS and ARC patients has been great. Long after they no longer require acute medical care, many AIDS/ ARC patients have remained hospitalized at a cost of over $400 per day (Whitlow 1988) because housing has been unavailable. Others have been unable to find housing after discharge. Because of their drug or alcohol abuse, family members are often unwilling or unable to house them, and they continue their addictive lifestyle until they return to the hospital.

In mid-1985, the New Jersey State Department of Health began working on solutions to this problem. The Post-Hospital Residential Program was developed to provide appropriate, cost-effective, posthospital placement for drug users who are homeless AIDS/ARC patients.

Four of New Jersey's residential drug treatment programs (therapeutic communities) were initially designated as pilot programs. Each facility was to house three patients at a reimbursement rate of $65.75 per bed per day, or $24,000 annually. This was significantly less than the estimated cost of staying in a hospital. The new residential program reimbursement rate was greater than the normal rate so that higher levels of medical, nursing, mental health, and social services could be provided for these patients. All personnel involved in this program were required to attend training sessions on the medical, psychiatric, and social service aspects of AIDS and ARC. Additional training is provided on a regular basis, and site visits are conducted regularly by

Department of Health personnel to review records and verify contract obligations.

To be admitted to this program, a patient must have a diagnosis of AIDS or ARC; (2) be ambulatory; (3) be independent in all activities of daily living; (4) be continent; (5) have clear mental status as certified by a psychiatrist; (6) be drug free or on methadone maintenance; and (7) be medically cleared for discharge from the acute care facility. All placements are coordinated and approved by the AIDS Community Support Unit office of the DNDAC to ensure that referrals are appropriate and meet requirements.

The Discharge Planner from the referral hospital must provide the AIDS Community Service Unit with a copy of the medical chart, along with the following information in the discharge treatment plan: (1) medication; (2) nutritional assessment with recommended diet plan; (3) complete psychological and social history; (4) a nursing plan; (5) all prescriptions; and (6) a medical appointment schedule. In addition, the referral hospital must include certification from a physician that the patient can be discharged to a residential facility and is not in need of higher levels of care, as well as documentation showing that application/referral for entitlement has been initiated by the hospital prior to placement. The hospital must agree to accept the patient when criteria for admission are no longer met. This information is transferred to the Drug Treatment Program when placement is made.

The Residential Treatment Facility is required to provide the following services:

(1)   medical assessment and referral--minimum of 1-hour physician contact per patient per week;

(2)   nursing assessment and liaison with treating hospital--RN daily contact to include nursing assessment, dietary supervision, and medication dispensing;

(3)   mental health services--M.A.-level therapist to provide individual, group, and family therapy and support services, and psychiatrist to be available for consultation;

(4)   transportation to medical and other services;

(5)   special medications and supplies;

(6)   regular drug treatment services modified as medically or psychi-
        atrically indicated; and

(7)   continuation of methadone treatment where medically indicated.

The residential programs have different characteristics (e.g.,
Spanish-speaking, geographic location), and attempts are made to
place the patient in the most appropriate program and to maximize
bed utilization. Programs interview potential residents for acceptability but must notify the Department of Health when, and explain
why, an applicant is not approved for admission. All terminations or
discharges must also be reported.

During the treatment process, these AIDS/ARC patients receive therapeutic community-type counseling intervention, so that their own
potentially harmful drug use is curtailed, as is behavior that might
transmit AIDS to others.

As of May 1987, 43 homeless AIDS/ARC drug abuse patients were
housed through the AIDS/ARC residential program for a total of 3,941
bed-days. The average length of stay was 93 days. The program has
been remarkably cost effective: The cost of maintaining these
patients at $65.75 per day was $267,000 vs. $1,576,000 if they had
remained in acute care. Originally, the AIDS/ARC residential program
was composed of 4 participating programs and 12 beds and quickly
expanded to 5 programs and 19 beds by 1987. As of July 1, 1988, the
AIDS/ARC residential program contracts for 35 residential beds.

There have been few reports of other residents showing anxiety or
leaving the program because of the admission of AIDS/ARC patients;
in fact, therapeutic communities report that other patients are for
the most part sympathetic and supportive and serve as family surrogates to these homeless patients. There have been occasional problems
with programs that are unwilling to modify their concepts and practices to accommodate the social, psychological, and pharmacological
needs of the AIDS patients. Referral sources have also caused problems by referring inappropriate patients, particularly those requiring
skilled nursing care, and by not providing necessary records. These
problems are dealt with individually and have decreased as the program continues.

This program is not a panacea for housing problems of AIDS patients,
as many AIDS/ARC patients who are drug abusers refuse to enter a
structured regimen. The AIDS/ARC Residential Program does,

however, provide a cost-effective, appropriate alternative to retaining AIDS/ARC patients who do not require acute care in hospital beds, and who are willing to accept structured therapeutic community treatment. The clinical impression is that longevity is enhanced for these patients; this issue is now under study.

Medical Day Care

In addition to the Post-Hospital Residential Placement Program, the New Jersey State Department of Health has developed Medical Day Care Units for drug abusers with AIDS/ARC who can be discharged from the hospital and reside with their families or "significant others." The AIDS/ARC Medical Day Care Program addresses the needs of recipients of the New Jersey Medicaid Program who could benefit from a health services alternative to institutionalization.

AIDS Medical Day Care is a program of medically supervised, health-related services provided in an ambulatory structured drug treatment program setting to persons who do not require 24-hour inpatient institutional care. Medical, nursing, social, transportation, personal care, dietary, recreational, rehabilitative, drug counseling, and dental care services are included. The program enables IVDU AIDS patients to remain in the community, in homes where they would be unattended during the day. The structured drug treatment setting is designed to help reduce drug use and provide a cost-effective, humane mode of health care. It is believed that the participants' own health maintenance will be supervised, and their transmission behavior reduced.

The first AIDS Medical Day Care Unit opened in April 1988. This program accommodates up to 20 AIDS patients per day, Monday through Friday.

CONCLUSION

Contrary to the traditional belief that substance abusers are generally uncooperative and/or unresponsive to their own well-being, no less society's welfare, public health AIDS education efforts in various States have successfully educated this most problematic AIDS risk group. Once educated, IVDUs have self-reported risk reduction behavioral changes in both unsafe drug use and sexual activities (Selwyn 1986; Des Jarlais et al. 1988). It is becoming clear to health care professionals across the Nation that IVDUs are reachable.

It is important to devote special attention to IVDUs not only to curtail further AIDS transmission within this population, but also to prevent the sexual and perinatal spread of AIDS. This effort must start with increased funding for various drug treatment services. The goal should be to encourage treatment admissions and to provide affordable, accessible care to all who can be persuaded to apply for it. The AIDS emergency demands that drug treatment programs extend their efforts to those addicts who do not enter treatment, with a public-health-oriented message to reduce transmission behaviors. Outreach efforts must expand to all groups of drug users, especially minority groups. Our experience indicates that treatment admissions are enhanced by such an approach, rather than reduced.

Many of the growing numbers of people with AIDS in New Jersey will depend upon public support for their medical and psychosocial needs. The care of each person with AIDS is estimated to cost tens of thousands of dollars over the course of the illness (New Jersey State Department of Health 1987a). To address the escalating demand for resources, the Federal Government, in collaboration with each State's medical and social service providers and their Departments of Health, must work together to develop innovative service system networks to care for people with AIDS. It is essential that these services are humane and cost effective.

The role of community-based drug treatment centers must expand to meet this public health emergency, as they are the only health care system with which large numbers of addicts voluntarily interact. They are in a position to provide consistent educational messages and support for behavioral change. Treatment programs can furnish the addicted population with primary medical care where other providers are scarce, overburdened, or unable to relate well to this population. They are able to afford symptomatic clients with case management and support services geared to their special needs. The nature and mixture of services will vary according to the infection rate and other characteristics of the addict population.

REFERENCES

Battjes, R.J. Personal communication, 1988.
Des Jarlais, D.C.; Friedman, S.R.; and Hopkins, W. Risk reduction for the acquired immunodeficiency syndrome among intravenous drug abusers. In: Galea, R.P.; Lewis, B.F.; and Baker, L.A., eds. *AIDS and IV Drug Abusers: Current Perspectives.* Owings Mills, MD: Rynd Communications, 1988. pp. 97-107.

French, J. New Jersey State Department of Health, Trenton. Personal communications, January 1988.

Ginzburg, H.M. Acquired immune deficiency syndrome and drug abuse. In: Galea, R.P.; Lewis, B.F.; and Baker, L.A., eds. *AIDS and IV Drug Abusers: Current Perspectives*. Owings Mills, MD: Rynd Communications, 1988. pp. 61-63.

Ginzburg, H.M.; French, J.; Jackson, J.; Hartsock, P.I.; MacDonald, M.G.; and Weiss, S.H. Health education and knowledge assessment of HTLV-III disease among intravenous drug users. *Health Educ Q* 13(4) Winter, 1986. pp. 377-379.

Jackson, J.F. Written Testimony: Presidential Commission on the HIV Epidemic. Paper presented at Washington, DC, December 18, 1987.

Jackson, J.F.; Rotkiewicz, L.G.; Quinones, M.A.; and Passannante, M.R. A coupon program: Drug treatment and AIDS education. *Int J Addict* 24, in press.

New Jersey State Department of Health. *Statistical Perspectives on Drug Abuse Treatment in New Jersey, 1984*. Trenton, June 1985. p. 1.

New Jersey State Department of Health. *Statistical Perspectives on Drug Abuse Treatment in New Jersey, 1985*. Trenton, November 1986. pp. 4, 10, 12.

New Jersey State Department of Health. *AIDS in New Jersey—A Report from the Department of Health*. Trenton, April 1987a. p. 6.

New Jersey State Department of Health. *AIDS Cases--State of New Jersey as of July 1, 1987-December 1, 1987*. Trenton, 1987b. 4 pp.

New Jersey State Department of Health. *AIDS Cases--State of New Jersey as of January 31, 1988*. Trenton, 1988. 4 pp.

Schadl, R. New Jersey State Department of Health, Trenton. Personal communication, February 1988.

Selwyn, P.A. *AIDS: What Is Now Known*. New York: HP Publishing Company, 1986. pp. 18, 19, 68.

Star-Ledger. AIDS toll forecast doubled. November 5, 1987. p. 1.

Weiss, S.; Ginzburg, H.; and Altman, R. Risk factors for HTLV-III/LAV infection and the development of AIDS among drug abusers in New Jersey. Paper presented at the Second International Conference on AIDS, Paris, June 1986.

Whitlow, J. '88 viewed as turning point for health institutions. *Star-Ledger*, January 24, 1988. p. 23.

AUTHORS

Joyce F. Jackson, M.A.
Director

Leslie G. Rotkiewicz, M.P.A., M.A.
Chief, Administration and Evaluation

Robert C. Baxter, M.P.A., M.Ed.
Clinical Operations Specialist

AIDS Community Support Unit
New Jersey State Department of Health
20 Evergreen Place, 2d Floor
East Orange, NJ 07018
(201) 414-4404

Lost Opportunity to Combat AIDS: Drug Abusers in the Criminal Justice System

Eric D. Wish, Joyce O'Neil, and Virginia Baldau

INTRODUCTION

In the absence of a cure for acquired immunodeficiency syndrome (AIDS), societal efforts are aimed toward limiting the spread of the disease. To accomplish this, information regarding the risk behaviors for contracting and transmitting the disease is being distributed to the general population. In addition, outreach programs are being established in many cities to identify subgroups of the community for AIDS education and counseling. Most of these programs have been directed toward drug abusers and homosexuals, persons whose behavior may place them at high risk for AIDS.

Persons who inject illicit drugs constitute the predominant source of heterosexual and perinatal transmission of the human immuno-deficiency virus (HIV) that leads to AIDS (Des Jarlais and Hunt 1988). Drug injectors are at high risk of AIDS because their needle-sharing behavior makes them vulnerable to HIV infection, which, in turn, they can spread: by exchanging body fluids; by sharing injection equipment; and, in the case of female drug users, by transmission from mother to infant.

Because persons do not generally publicize their injection of illicit drugs, AIDS outreach programs typically locate drug injectors by approaching persons who have entered publicly funded treatment programs, or by establishing bases in minority neighborhoods known to be frequented by drug abusers. This paper suggests that an important additional avenue exists for reaching drug injectors—by approaching the thousands of drug abusers among arrestees and persons supervised by the criminal justice system.

Data from the Drug Use Forecasting (DUF) System of the National Institute of Justice (NIJ) (DUF Statistics 1988) has documented the high prevalence of recent illicit drug use by arrestees in the largest U.S. cities. For example, the prevalence of recent cocaine use, measured by urinalysis, is about 10 times that found in interview surveys of student and household populations. In addition, the majority of drug injectors surveyed through DUF indicated that they had injected cocaine. Since other injectable drugs like meth-amphetamines and opiates were also detected in various regions of the country, one might expect that the offender population would contain substantial numbers of drug injectors at risk for AIDS.

To assess the potential risk of HIV infection in offenders, this report analyzes new information from DUF interviews about drug injection and needle-sharing behaviors in male and female arrestees. Because female arrestees may be at special risk of AIDS--females tend to have more serious drug abuse problems than females and are likely to engage in prostitution with numerous partners (Goldstein 1979; Wish et al. 1985; Des Jarlais et al. 1987), this chapter focuses special attention on female arrestees.

THE DUF PROGRAM

In 1987, the NIJ established the DUF program, a national data system for tracking drug use trends in arrestees. Every 3 months, a new sample of approximately 250 male arrestees in each participating city is asked to agree to a voluntary and anonymous interview about their drug abuse and treatment history and to provide a voluntary urine specimen for analysis. Arrestees are usually interviewed soon after arrest in the city's central booking facility. Urine specimens are tested by Enzyme Multiplied Immune Test (EMIT) technology for 10 drugs: opiates, cocaine, PCP, marijuana, amphetamines (all positives are confirmed by gas chroma- tography), methadone, Darvon, barbiturates, methaqualone, and Valium. (The latter five drugs have rarely been found in the DUF samples.)

DUF interviewers intentionally oversample males charged with serious nondrug crimes because it is already well established that persons charged with the sale or possession of drugs are likely to be users (Wish and Johnson 1986). Because the resulting DUF samples have a smaller proportion of persons charged with drug offenses than would be found in a random sample of arrestees, DUF estimates of drug use should be viewed as minimum estimates of recent drug use in all arrestees.

DUF interviewers typically station themselves in each city's booking facility for 14 consecutive evenings during the busiest shifts. Over 90 percent of arrestees who are approached agree to be interviewed, and about 85 percent of the interviewees provide a voluntary urine specimen. DUF is currently operating in 13 cities: New York; Washington, DC; Portland, OR; San Diego, CA; Indianapolis, IN; Houston, TX; Fort Lauderdale, FL; Detroit, MI; New Orleans, LA; Phoenix, AZ; Chicago, IL; Los Angeles, CA; and Dallas, TX.

In late 1987, five DUF sites began to collect information from female arrestees. Because the number of females arrested is typically far below that of males, DUF interviewers approached all available female arrestees, regardless of charge, during the 2-week data collection period. The goal was to interview and obtain urine specimens from 100 females in each city, every 3 months.

METHOD

Sample

The findings in this report come from the five sites that have obtained data from male and female arrestees: Los Angeles, San Diego, Phoenix, New Orleans, and New York City (Manhattan). The data were collected between September and December 1987. Response rates for each site appear in table 1.

Interview response rates for males ranged from 92 percent to 100 percent and from 89 percent to 100 percent for females. Between 81 percent and 95 percent of male interviewees and 70 percent to 96 percent of female interviewees provided a urine specimen for analysis. The resulting sample of arrestees from the five sites who were interviewed and provided a urine specimen contained 516 females and 991 males. (For this presentation, most of the following analyses aggregate information across the five sites. Some of the more significant findings are presented separately for each site to examine whether the findings apply to all cities.)

Demographic and Case Characteristics of Male and Female Arrestees

Table 2 presents descriptive information obtained from the arrest report and DUF interview for both males and females. Age distributions were quite similar for males and females with the modal age range being between 21 and 25 years old. Ethnicity was also similar

189

TABLE 1. *Percentage of male and female arrestees who agreed to be interviewed and who gave a urine specimen*

	San Diego		Los Angeles		Phoenix		New Orleans		New York	
	M	F	M	F	M	F	M	F	M	F
(Number Approached)	(231)	(77)	(278)	(206)	(205)	(102)	(199)	(104)	(247)	(129)
Agreed to Interview	98%	99%	97%	98%	100%	100%	100%	99%	92%	89%
Gave a Urine Specimen	84%	70%	81%	85%	95%	96%	94%	89%	90%	89%

in the two groups. The largest group of male and female arrestees were black. More than one-third (35 percent) of the female arrestees were white and more than a quarter of the male arrestees were Hispanic.

While larceny and drug offenses were the most common charges at arrest for both males and females, there were some differences between the two groups. Males were more likely to be charged with burglary (13 percent vs. 6 percent) or robbery (7 percent vs. 1 percent), while females were more likely to be charged with sex offenses, primarily prostitution (22 percent vs. 3 percent). Male arrestees' greater involvement in more serious crimes (seriousness as defined by legal statute) is evident in the finding that more males were charged with a felony offense (76 percent vs. 42 percent). This difference is also attributable to the fact, noted above, that females charged with felony offenses were not oversampled as males were. These differences in crime severity should not bias findings with regard to drug abuse. Moreover, prior studies have documented the diversity of crimes committed by drug abusers and indicate that the likelihood of testing positive at arrest is generally unrelated to the seriousness of the arrest charge (Wish et al. 1981; Wish and Johnson 1986).

TABLE 2. *Demographic and case characteristics of male and female arrestees*

	Percent of Males (n=991)	Percent of Females (n=516)
Age at Arrest		
15-20	17	12
21-25	29	30
26-30	21	27
31-35	14	16
36+	19	15
Ethnicity		
Black	41	45
White	29	35
Hispanic	28	18
Other	2	2
Top Charge at Arrest		
Larceny	15	18
Drug sale/possession	13	17
Burglary	13	6
Assault	10	7
Stolen property	10	4
Robbery	7	1
Weapons	4	*
Sex offense	3	22
Homicide/manslaughter	2	*
Other	23	23
Current Arrest a Felony	76	42

* = Less than 1 percent.

Limitations

Several limitations should be kept in mind when reviewing these findings. First, data about drug injection and needle sharing are based upon voluntary self-reports. Although every effort is made to convince arrestees of their anonymity and that the information cannot be used against them, the jail environment is inherently threatening, and there is considerable underreporting of recent illicit behaviors. It should be noted that many more persons test positive for drugs than admit to recent drug use in the interview. On the other hand, there is considerable internal consistency in the interview information from arrestees, and, when persons do report illicit behaviors, the information appears valid (Wish, in press). Because some arrestees do conceal their illegal behaviors, findings about injection and needle sharing should be viewed as minimal estimates of these behaviors in the arrestee population.

A second limitation involves the generalizability of these findings. In the pilot phase of DUF, we attempted to determine whether samples of 200 arrestees yielded estimates of drug use similar to those obtained by testing several thousand arrestees from the same city. We found that, in New York and in the District of Columbia, the estimates from the smaller samples were quite close (within 10 percentage points) to those from larger samples. We are less sure that our findings from the smaller samples of female arrestees (sometimes as low as 50 per city) are equally representative of the wider population of female arrestees in that jurisdiction. New data from female arrestees not included in this paper, however, have replicated the principal findings in this report. Finally, it should be noted that these findings apply to persons who have been arrested; they should not be generalized to the nonoffender population.

FINDINGS AND DISCUSSION

Urinalysis Results

Table 3 compares urinalysis results for the male and female arrestees in each of the five cities. In four of the cities (all except New Orleans), female arrestees were as likely to test positive for any of the 10 drugs as male arrestees. However, there were differences in the specific drugs detected in male and female arrestees. Females tended to be more likely to test positive for cocaine or heroin (opiates). The differences in heroin positives were especially large for arrestees in San Diego and in Phoenix. Marijuana was the one drug that appeared to be less prevalent in females. In Los Angeles, San Diego, and New Orleans only about half as many females as males tested positive for marijuana. Subsequent results from male and female arrestees tested in January through March 1988 replicated the above findings regarding the higher prevalence of cocaine and

192

TABLE 3. *Percentage of male and female arrestees who tested positive for drug use*

	DUF City	Percent of Males	Percent of Females
Positive for Any Drug	Los Angeles	69	80
	San Diego	75	87
	Phoenix	53	69
	New Orleans	72	46
	New York	79	83
Positive for Cocaine	Los Angeles	46	65
	San Diego	44	58
	Phoenix	21	36
	New Orleans	45	30
	New York	63	70
Positive for Opiates	Los Angeles	15	18
	San Diego	24	42
	Phoenix	5	14
	New Orleans	6	4
	New York	26	35
Positive for Marijuana	Los Angeles	28	8
	San Diego	44	24
	Phoenix	42	40
	New Orleans	48	25
	New York	28	25

heroin and lower prevalence of marijuana in female arrestees (DUF Statistics 1988).

These findings indicate that female arrestees are more involved with hard drugs such as heroin and cocaine than are male arrestees. They are consistent with results from a study of jailed arrestees in the 1970s (Wish et al. 1985) and a 1984 study of males and females arrested in Manhattan (Wish et al. 1986a). Because heroin and cocaine are often injected, these findings suggest that injection might be a more common behavior in female arrestees.

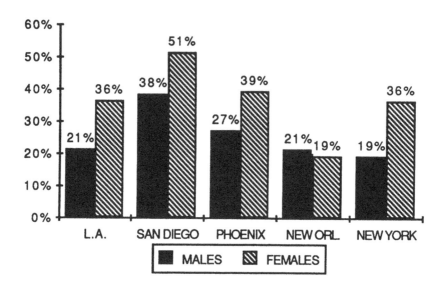

FIGURE 1. *Percent of male and female arrestees who ever injected (n=1,507)*

Drug Injection in Female Arrestees

Figure 1 shows the percentage of male and female arrestees who reported ever having injected drugs. In all cities except New Orleans, female arrestees were more likely to admit to injecting drugs. The largest differences were found in Los Angeles (36 percent vs. 21 percent) and New York (36 percent vs. 19 percent).

When factors that might be associated with drug injection in the females were examined (table 4), as expected, age was strongly associated with injection. While about one-fourth of the female arrestees under age 21 indicated having ever injected drugs, almost one-half (47 percent) of the women above age 30 had injected. Persons who had dropped out of school by the 10th grade also had a high rate of injection (50 percent). It should be noted that these dropouts are the very people whom school-based surveys and in-school AIDS prevention efforts would miss. However, there was little variation in injection by charge at arrest, except that persons charged with assault were least likely (18 percent) to have injected drugs. This is

194

TABLE 4. *Correlates of injection of female arrestees*

Correlate	(n)	Percent Ever Injected
Age at Arrest		
15-20	(60)	23
21-25	(154)	31
26-30	(139)	35
31+	(154)	47
Years of Education		
9 or less	(82)	50
10-11	(131)	37
12	(172)	26
13+	(111)	37
Ethnicity		
White	(176)	55
Hispanic	(90)	36
Black	(225)	22
Top Charge at Arrest		
Stolen property	(22)	50
Sex offenses	(115)	40
Burglary	(31)	39
Larceny	(95)	36
Drug sale/poss.	(87)	32
Assault	(34)	18
Other	(132)	36

consistent with previous research showing that assaulters are among those least likely to test positive for hard drugs at arrest (Wish et al. 1986a). Persons charged with sex offenses were not more likely to have injected drugs than persons charged with other types of offenses. However, some females charged with nonsex offenses may have engaged in prostitution at some time in their lives.

Ethnic Differences in Injection Practices

While it was expected that older females and school dropouts would be at a higher risk of drug injection, the extent of ethnic differences

in drug injection was surprising. White female arrestees were twice
as likely as black females to have injected drugs (55 percent vs.
22 percent, p<.001). Hispanic females were midway between these two
groups (36 percent). However, their small number, n=90, prohibits
further analysis of Hispanic females. If white females were more
likely to be older or to have dropped out of school, it might explain
why they had higher rates of injection. These factors, however, did
not account for the ethnic differences in injection.

Figure 2 shows that, in each of the five cities, white females were
more likely to have injected drugs. White female arrestees in San
Diego and Phoenix were twice as likely to report injection, and in
Los Angeles there was a threefold difference (72 percent vs.
20 percent).

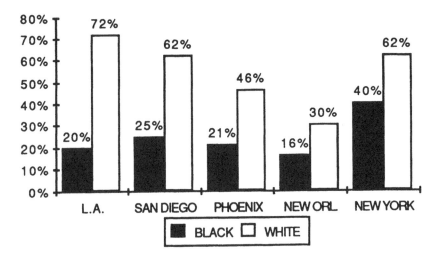

FIGURE 2. *Percent of female arrestees who ever injected,
by ethnicity (n=401)*

To investigate these ethnic differences in drug injection, we examined
other information from the DUF interview and test results. As sus-
pected, white females were twice as likely as black females (48 percent vs. 22 percent, p<.001) to report having been dependent on
heroin (table 5). No differences were found with regard to dependence on cocaine, however. In spite of their greater dependence on
heroin, white females were not more likely to report having received

TABLE 5. *Heroin and cocaine use and dependence in female arrestees, by ethnicity*

Drug Use	Percent Black (n=225)	Percent White (n=176)
Self Reports		
Ever dependent on heroin	22	48
Ever dependent on cocaine	22	23
Ever received drug treatment	23	30
Urine Test at Arrest		
Positive for heroin	10	27
Positive for cocaine	60	47

drug abuse treatment (30 percent vs. 23 percent, not a statistically significant difference).

These differences could have occurred if white arrestees had been more willing than black arrestees to report illicit behaviors to the interviewer. Attempts were made to minimize such a bias by ensuring that the ethnic composition of DUF interviewers was similar to that of the arrestees in each city. Furthermore, the urine test results supported the interview findings. White female arrestees were almost three times as likely to test positive for heroin than were black females (27 percent vs. 10 percent, p<.001). Black females were more likely to test positive for cocaine (60 percent vs. 47 percent, p<.05). However, white female cocaine users were three times more likely to report a preference for injecting cocaine than were black female cocaine users (40 percent vs. 13 percent, respectively, p<.001). Black females who used cocaine said they typically preferred to smoke, freebase, or snort the drug.

Figure 3 shows the urine test results for heroin for black and white arrestees. In every city, white female arrestees were more likely to test positive for heroin. The largest differences were found in Los Angeles, Phoenix, and New Orleans, where white females were more than three times as likely to test positive for heroin than were black females.

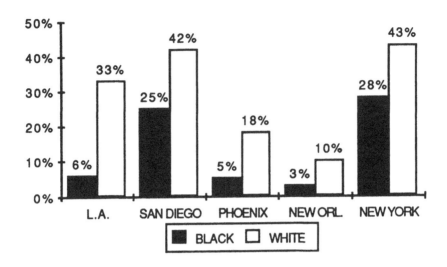

FIGURE 3. *Percent of female arrestees who tested positive for opiates, by ethnicity*

These findings suggest that there is both a greater involvement of white females in heroin and a reluctance on the part of black females to inject drugs. Even when black females reported using cocaine, they tended to take the drug through routes other than injection. A similar finding of more intravenous heroin use by white females than by black females has also been reported in a study of females admitted to methadone maintenance programs and therapeutic communities in five cities (Moise et al. 1982).

Deviance and Drug Abuse Practices

Some authors have suggested a concept of relative deviance that may explain why white female arrestees may be more serious drug abusers (Dembo and Shern 1982). According to this theory, persons who aremore deviant from the norms of their social and cultural setting will exhibit more serious behavior problems and psychopathology (Kaufman 1978). White females are typically a small proportion of all arrested females and could be expected to be more deviant than black females. While this hypothesis cannot be tested directly, the level of deviance was measured.

Age of initiation of drug use is generally considered to be a strong correlate of deviance. The younger a person is when she begins to use drugs, the more likely she is to proceed to dysfunctional drug abuse and other behavior problems. If white female arrestees were more heavily involved with drugs, we would expect them to have begun to use and inject drugs earlier. Table 6 shows this to be the case.

White females were likely to begin the use of alcohol, heroin, and marijuana about 2 years earlier than black females who were arrested. They began to use cocaine 3 years earlier than black arrestees. The median age of first drug injection was about 4 years earlier in white females than in black females. In addition, the ages of onset for Hispanic females, not presented here, were virtually identical to those of the black females.

TABLE 6. *Median age of onset of drug use and injection in black and white female arrestees (arrestees from five DUF sites)*

	White Females	Black Females
First Tried Marijuana	13+	15+
First Tried Alcohol	14+	16+
First Tried Heroin	17+	19
First Injected	17+	21+
First Tried Cocaine	18+	21+

These findings, together with the urinalysis results, offer strong evidence that white female arrestees are among the most serious drug abusers in the arrestee population. Their drug injection puts them at high risk for contracting and transmitting HIV.

Needle-Sharing Behaviors and AIDS

If a person reported injecting drugs, additional questions were asked about needle sharing. Few differences were found between male and female injectors with regard to sharing needles, although there were some regional differences (table 7). Almost one-half of male and

TABLE 7. *Needle-sharing behavior in male and female drug injectors*

	Los Angeles		San Diego		Phoenix		New Orleans		New York	
	M	F	M	F	M	F	M	F	M	F
Injectors Who Share	47%	50%	27%	26%	37%	32%	23%	18%	5%	24%
Sharers Who Changed Because of AIDS	78%	68%	47%	59%	63%	76%	90%	78%	95%	50%

female injectors in Los Angeles said that they currently shared their needles with one or more persons. In the rest of the country, the percentage was closer to 20 to 25 percent. New York male injectors were least likely to admit sharing needles (5 percent), although interviewers for this study said that male arrestees were uncomfortable about this topic and probably underreported needle sharing.

The majority of both male and female arrestees who shared needles after learning about AIDS stated they had changed their behaviors in some way because of the AIDS epidemic. Almost all male sharers interviewed in New Orleans and New York indicated that they had changed their needle-sharing behaviors. This did not necessarily imply that their altered behaviors were effective in reducing their vulnerability to AIDS.

The interviewers recorded verbatim each respondent's explanation for why and how they had or had not changed their behaviors as a result of AIDS. Several of these unedited comments appear in table 8. While male and female arrestees claimed they were taking steps to avoid AIDS, their answers underscored a number of misconceptions regarding the disease. For example, a comment frequently made was that individuals shared needles only with persons who did not look sick. This is an ineffective strategy for avoiding infection because HIV has a long incubation period and infected persons may have no symptoms for several years.

TABLE 8. *How has AIDS changed your needle-sharing behavior?*
(Unedited responses from arrestees in five cities)

Males

"Don't share needles with anyone who partakes in homosexual activities." (Los Angeles - Id#3228)

"You can tell if a person is clean and keeps themselves together. Don't share with unclean people." (Los Angeles - Id#3208)

If sharing, cleans with water - usually uses needle first. (San Diego - Id#850)

Cleans with more care - bleach; shares less - change works more often. (San Diego - Id#804)

"AIDS has caused me to slow down on needle sharing, but not stop completely." (Phoenix - Id#209)

Sharing is *"dependent upon specific circumstances. If necessary, will share."* (Phoenix - Id#102)

"I shared my works because we only had one, and I just take a chance and hope not to get AIDS. As many as five people share the same needle. There is no limit to the amount of people that can use the same needle." (New Orleans - Id#577)

"I never worry about getting AIDS because of using the same needles with my friends." (New Orleans - Id#588)

"Only share with people I know or in case of emergency." (New York - Id#3034)

Shares *"a little, still shares with friends."* (New York - Id#3043)

Females

"I don't think I can get it. I don't think the people I do it with have it." (Los Angeles - Id#4049)

"Don't share as much. Share with just one person." Cleans with alcohol. (Los Angeles - Id#4003)

Has found it difficult to get needles. *"Use whatever needles I can find."* Aware of AIDS and still shares. (San Diego - Id#2041)

"Only inject by myself. Before shared with friends." (San Diego - Id#2085)

"Needles are easier to buy so there is no needle sharing at present." (Phoenix - Id#262)

"Quit sharing needles due to AIDS scare." (Phoenix - Id#294)

"It doesn't matter if I share them or not as long as I get my drugs." (New Orleans - Id#594)

TABLE 8. (Continued)

---

*"Because I only had a few needles so we shared. I didn't want to sit
    there and see everyone else doing it."* (New Orleans - Id#703)
"I only share with one person - my boyfriend, and he is clean."
    (New York - Id#3161)
"I share because there are no works at the gallery."
    (New York - Id#3290)

Responses from male and female arrestees frequently demonstrated a
fear of AIDS and a desire to avoid infection. Arrestees and other
criminal justice system detainees therefore are a receptive audience
for education, prevention, and treatment programs. An invaluable
opportunity exists to correct their misconceptions about AIDS.

SUMMARY AND POLICY IMPLICATIONS

Summary

There is a critical need to identify persons who are likely to inject
drugs, so that they can be taught to limit the spread of AIDS. Results from the DUF program indicate that more than 50 percent of
arrestees in large cities in the United States test positive for illicit
drugs. If many of these persons also inject drugs, a special opportunity to reach persons at high risk for AIDS may be available.

New information from DUF interviews about drug injection and needle
sharing in male and female arrestees in five cities was analyzed to
examine the characteristics of female drug injectors. The findings
indicated that, while illicit drug use is prevalent in all arrestees,
females are more likely to test positive for injectable drugs like
heroin or cocaine and are more likely to report having injected
drugs. By the time these women passed age 30, about one-half had
injected a drug. About one-half of the females who dropped out of
school had also injected drugs.

Dramatic ethnic differences were found in injection behavior of
females. White females were most likely to have injected drugs.
This difference was partially explained by the fact that white females
were more seriously involved with heroin. Differences in drugs used,
however, could not completely account for the ethnic differences in
injection. Even though black and white female arrestees appeared to

202

be similarly involved with cocaine, white women were far more likely to inject cocaine.

Other researchers have found similar ethnic differences in injection practices of female drug abusers. One hypothesis is that white females who are involved with hard drugs or who are arrested in the United States tend to be more deviant. As expected, white females did have an earlier age of onset of drug use and began to inject drugs about 4 years earlier than black females. This apparent deviance, drug abuse, and involvement in prostitution puts female arrestees, especially white female arrestees, at unusually high risk for AIDS.

Needle sharing was reported by one-quarter to one-half of both male and female arrestees interviewed. The majority of male and female sharers did indicate, however, that they had changed their needle-sharing behaviors as a result of the AIDS epidemic. Unfortunately, misconceptions about AIDS were common. Thus, some of the precautions that they were taking, such as sharing only with someone who did not look sick, were ineffective and gave a false sense of security. The sensitivity and responsiveness of the arrestees to the AIDS problem, along with their apparent ignorance of the best methods to avoid the disease, suggest that it might be possible to reduce the spread of AIDS by initiating education, prevention, and treatment programs for arrestees.

Policy Implications

Although these findings are from arrestees, there is ample evidence that incarcerated persons and those released on probation or parole are a subset of the arrestee population with serious drug problems (Wish and Johnson 1986; Wish et al. 1986b). Thus, all persons detained or supervised by the criminal justice system should be considered at much greater risk of illicit drug use and AIDS than is the general population.

Although we did not test any of our samples of arrestees for the presence of antibodies to HIV, estimates of seropositivity rates in drug injectors are available from other sources. The rates vary considerably across the country from less than 5 percent of drug injectors in New Orleans and Los Angeles to over 50 percent for injectors in New York City and northern New Jersey (Des Jarlais and Hunt 1988). Using the estimate of 50 percent seropositive drug injectors in New York City, and DUF statistics showing that about 25 percent

(19 percent of males and 36 percent of females) of all arrestees in New York have ever injected drugs, we project that at least 12,500 of the 100,000 persons arrested in Manhattan each year (25 percent x 100,000 x 50 percent) would test positive for HIV. This may be an underestimate, because the DUF program undersampled persons charged with drug offenses, and an unknown percentage of arrestees refused to admit to injecting drugs.

Because of the high seropositivity rates in New York City drug injectors, the estimates above should not be applied directly to arrestees in other cities. It is not known whether drug abusers in other cities will eventually develop rates of seropositivity similar to drug injectors in New York. Mass screening programs of the general population of prison inmates across the country have generally reported rates of seropositivity below 3 percent, but one sample of "high-risk" inmates, defined as homosexuals or drug injectors, in Houston found that 33 percent of those tested were seropositive (Hammett 1988). Consistent with this study, epidemiological surveys of inmates in Maryland correctional facilities between 1985 and 1987 found that females had twice the seropositivity rate as males (15 percent vs. 7 percent). These seropositivity rates in prison inmates are somewhat lower than expected from the rates of drug injection found in this study. As suggested below, however, there are reasons to believe that inmate populations may contain fewer active street criminal drug abusers who show up repeatedly in the arrestee population.

By definition, criminal justice system detainees are readily accessible to societal efforts to modify the behaviors that increase their risk for AIDS. Unfortunately, the enormity of the opportunity for treating these persons contrasts greatly with the paucity of efforts devoted to this task.

To be sure, all State and Federal prisons and most large city jails provide AIDS information and training (Hammett 1988). These institutions have been quick to respond to the AIDS epidemic because they have to house persons for long periods of time and are therefore more vulnerable to problems stemming from infected residents. Thus, staff or inmate training programs are available in jails or prisons where persons are detained for some time. In contrast, the much larger population of arrestees and probationers, who are typically released back in to the community, are less likely to receive AIDS information. In establishing the DUF program in the largest booking facilities in the country, interview staff have not seen a single AIDS education or counseling program for arrestees. Arrestees in the major cities of this country tend to be housed for hours (before arraignment) in large pens with no attempts to intervene for drug abuse.

A recent survey of probation and parole departments in all 50 States found that less than half (about 40 percent) have education, prevention, or information programs for persons being released to the community (Hunt 1988). Most of the departments with a program simply hand out public health or Red Cross brochures about AIDS that are not expressly tailored to the education level and needs of offenders returning to the community. The majority of these departments provide this limited information only to persons believed to have a high risk for AIDS (persons charged with sex offenses, known drug injectors, and homosexuals). This strategy could miss many drug abusers (and their sexual partners) because criminal justice records and arrest or conviction charges are poor indicators of drug abuse.

The interviewers also found that, although probation and parole departments included in the study expressed a "desperate" interest in providing expanded AIDS programs for releasees, they were hampered by inadequate funds and a lack of available trained personnel. Their report recommended that mandatory AIDS training be provided for all staff and for all probationers and parolees (Hunt 1988).

By failing to focus sufficient resources on addressing the drug abuse and AIDS problem in arrestees and probationers, the country is losing an important opportunity to reach the largest pool of serious drug abusers entering the criminal justice system. Because of the extensive overcrowded conditions in the Nation's jails, there is a deliberate attempt to detain as few arrestees as possible. Persons charged with many of the more common petty offenses committed by drug abusers (larcenies, lesser drug offenses, and prostitution) are routinely released back to the community soon after arrest (pending trial) or, if convicted, receive a fine, time served (the time already detained before disposition satisfies the sentence), or a term of probation (Johnson et al. 1985). Some of these street criminals may be detained overnight in jails but rarely are sentenced to prison, where most of the AIDS programs exist. It is this large group of arrestees and probationers, who return to their drug-abusing friends and sexual partners, for whom AIDS education and drug abuse treatment is most crucial.

Unfortunately, with one exception, systematic identification of drug-abusing arrestees and referral to treatment is rare. It should be noted that DUF is an anonymous program. Only the District of Columbia has a fully operational program to test all arrestees for drug use by urinalysis. Six participating jurisdictions are currently being funded by the Bureau of Justice Assistance to replicate the District's pretrial testing program and are at varying stages of development. Persons who test positive are referred by the judge to urine monitoring and/or treatment programs as a condition of pretrial release (Carver 1986). Although probation (and parole) officers have the authority to order drug tests for persons they supervise, few departments have the resources to screen all persons for drug use. Without drug testing, most drug abusers in the criminal justice system avoid detection (Wish 1988).

Nonanonymous drug testing has the advantage of enabling the identification of persons to be referred to treatment programs or AIDS counseling, but is costly and takes time to develop. Still, there are a number of other relatively inexpensive strategies that can be rapidly adopted. Every person arrested or under the supervision of the criminal justice system could be presented with educational information about prevention of AIDS. Posters informing persons about the risk behaviors for AIDS and listing drug abuse treatment referral and AIDS information sources could be displayed in every police station, booking facility, probation and parole office, and detention center across the country. For example, credible AIDS videotapes could be shown once an hour to the "captive audiences" in urban booking facilities. It seems that if only a small subset of the detainees listened to the information, it would still be beneficial. Clearly, this information will have to be developed for diverse reading levels and language problems. It has also been suggested that some of these programs be directed toward the spouses and sexual partners of probationers and parolees (Hunt 1988).

In view of their exceptional risk for drug injection and perinatal transmission of AIDS, female arrestees could receive individual counseling about how to avoid the disease. If trained justice personnel are not available, local health departments could be requested to station trained personnel in central booking facilities. The relatively small number of females who are arrested, even in the largest cities, makes individual counseling a feasible approach.

Our findings also suggest that outreach and prevention programs both inside and outside the criminal justice system should not be limited to members of minority groups. These programs should also be provided for deviant white females who have been arrested or who are likely to be committing crimes or abusing drugs.

Although further research is needed to determine which of the above strategies will be most effective, the magnitude of the drug abuse and AIDS problems in persons entering the criminal justice system presents a compelling case for immediate action.

REFERENCES

Carver, J.A. Drugs and crime: Controlling use and reducing risk through testing. *NIJ Reports* 199, September 1986.

Dembo, R., and Shern, D. Relative deviance and the process of drug involvement among inner-city youths. *Int J Addict* 17:1373-1399, 1982.

Des Jarlais, D., and Hunt, D. AIDS and intravenous drug use. *NIJ AIDS Bulletin.* U.S. Department of Justice, February 1988. p. 6.

Des Jarlais, D.J.; Wish, E.D.; Friedman, S.R.; Stoneburner, R.; Yancovitz, S.R.; Mildvan, D.; El-Sadr, W.; Brady, E.; and Cuadrado, M. Intravenous drug use and the heterosexual transmission of the human immunodeficiency virus—current trends in New York City. *NY State J Med* 87:283-285, 1987.

DUF Statistics, January 1988. Washington, DC: National Institute of Justice.

DUF Statistics, May, 1988. Washington, DC: National Institute of Justice.

Goldstein, P. *Prostitution and Drugs.* Lexington, MA: Lexington Books, 1979. 190 pp.

Hammett, T.M. *AIDS in Correctional Facilities: Issues and Options.* 3rd ed. Washington, DC: National Institute of Justice, 1988. p. 28.

Hunt, D. *AIDS in Community Corrections: Issues and Options.* Washington, DC: National Institute of Justice, 1988. p. 107.

Johnson, B.D.; Goldstein, P.J.; Preble, E.; Schmeidler, J.; Lipton, D.; Spunt, B.; and Miller, T. *Taking Care of Business: The Economics of Crime by Heroin Abusers.* Lexington, MA: Lexington Books, 1985. 278 pp.

Kaufman, E. The relationship of social class and ethnicity to drug abuse. In: Smith, D.E.; Anderson, S.M.; Buxton, M.; Gottlieb, N.; Harvey, W.; and Chung, T., eds. *A Multicultural View of Drug Abuse.* Cambridge, MA: Shenkman, 1978. pp. 158-164.

Moise, R.; Kovach, J.; Reed, B.; and Bellows, N. A comparison of black and white women entering drug abuse treatment programs. *Int J Addict* 17:35–49, 1982.

Wish, E.D. Urine testing of criminals: What are we waiting for? *J Policy Anal Mgmt* 7:551-554, 1988.

Wish, E.D. Identifying drug abusing criminals. In: Leukefeld, C., and Tims, F. *Compulsory Treatment of Drug Abuse: Research and Clinical Practice.* National Institute on Drug Abuse Research Monograph 86. DHHS Pub. No. (ADM) 88-1578. Washington, DC: Supt. of Docs., U.S. Govt. Print. Off., 1988. pp. 139-159.

Wish, E.D.; Brady, E.; Cuadrado, M.; and Alvarado, L. Female arrestees: The most serious drug abusers? Presented at the Annual Meeting of the American Society of Criminology, San Diego, CA, November 1985.

Wish, E.D.; Brady, E.; and Cuadrado, M. Urine testing of arrestees: Findings from Manhattan. Presented at the National Institute of Justice-sponsored conference, "Drugs and Crime: Detecting Use and Reducing Risk." Washington DC, June 5, 1986a.

Wish, E.D.; Cuadrado, M.; and Martorana, J. Estimates of drug use in intensive supervision probationers: Results from a pilot study. *Federal Probation.* Vol. 4. December, 1986b.

Wish, E.D., and Johnson, B.D. The impact of substance abuse on criminal careers. In: Blumstein, A.; Cohen, J.; Roth, J.; and Visher, C.A., eds. *Criminal Careers and Career Criminals.* Vol. II. Washington, DC: National Academy Press, 1986. pp. 52-88.

Wish, E.D.; Klumpp, K.A.; Moorer, A.H.; Brady, E.; and Williams, K.M. *An Analysis of Drugs and Crime Among Arrestees in the District of Columbia. Executive Summary.* (U.S. Department of Justice) Washington, DC: Supt. of Docs., , U.S. Govt. Print. Off., December 1981.

ACKNOWLEDGMENT

This work was supported by Visiting Fellow grant 87-IJ-CX-0008 from the National Institute of Justice, U.S. Department of Justice.

AUTHORS

Eric D. Wish, Ph.D.
Joyce O'Neil, M.A.
Virginia Baldau, B.A.

Department of Justice
National Institute of Justice
633 Indiana Avenue, N.W.
Washington, DC 20530

The Homeless Intravenous Drug Abuser and the AIDS Epidemic

Herman Joseph and Hilda Roman-Nay

INTRODUCTION

The topics addressed in this chapter deal with interrelationships among three of the most pressing contemporary social and public health issues confronting American society: homelessness, intravenous (IV) drug abuse, and the acquired immunodeficiency syndrome (AIDS) epidemic. Homelessness and IV drug abuse affect each other, and each must be addressed if the AIDS epidemic is to be curtailed and contained. The uncertainties inherent in a state of homelessness prevent most homeless IV drug users (IVDUs) from adopting adequate and sustained risk reduction behavior to avoid transmitting or contracting AIDS. Furthermore, the state of homelessness makes delivery of effective medical and social services a tenuous undertaking at best. This paper will summarize the extent of the problem, describe a number of surveys and exploratory studies of the population, and present examples of programs that affect homeless IVDUs and the AIDS epidemic.

EXTENT OF THE PROBLEM

Extent of the AIDS Epidemic in New York City

Of the 53,069 AIDS cases in the United States reported to the Centers for Disease Control (CDC) as of February 1988, 13,401 (25 percent) were reported from New York City. Table 1 presents the number of adult AIDS cases in New York City by risk factor by race by sex as of February 24, 1988. The data were compiled by the AIDS surveillance unit of the New York City Department of Health (1988a).

210

TABLE 1. *AIDS risk groups by race by sex*

	Males					
Risk Category	Black	White	His- panic	Other*	Total	(%)
Sex with Man at Risk	1,340	4,611	1,132	60	7,143	(61)
Sex with Man at Risk/IV	219	234	164	2	619	(5)
IV Drug Use	1,448	483	1,351	7	3,289	(28)
Persons from Countries Where Risks Are Unclear	209	0	0	0	209	(2)
Sex Partner of Woman at Risk	4	3	1	0	8	(1)
Transfusion	10	40	5	3	58	(1)
Blood Products	1	19	2	0	22	(1)
No Identified Risk	19	11	21	3	34	(1)
Other**	93	48	89	7	237	(2)
Total (%)	3,343 211(29)	5,549 (47)	2,765 (24)	82 (1)	11,639	

* Includes 69 Asians, 8 Native Americans, and persons for whom race/ethnicity is not known.

** Includes persons who died before interview, who refused investigation or whose doctor refused, and persons still under investigation for risk.

SOURCE: New York City Department of Health (1988a).

TABLE 1. (Continued)

Risk Category	Females					
	Black	White	His-panic	Other*	Total	(%)
IV Drug Abuse	456	137	282	1	876	(59)
Persons from Countries Where Risks Are Unclear	53	0	0	0	53	(4)
Sex Partner of Man at Risk	137	51	144	1	333	(22)
Transfusion	18	27	144	1	55	(1)
Blood Products	1	0	0	0	1	(1)
No Identified Risk	17	7	7	0	31	(2)
Other**	85	22	32	1	140	(9)
Totals (%)	767 (51)	244 (16)	474 (32)	4 (1)	1,489	
Total Male and Female (%)	4,110 (31)	5,693 (43)	3,239 (25)	80 (1)	13,128	

* Includes 69 Asians, 8 Native Americans, and persons for whom race/ethnicity is not known.

** Includes persons who died before interview, who refused investigation or whose doctor refused, and persons still under investigation for risk.

SOURCE: New York City Department of Health (1988a).

These statistics indicate that patterns of risk behavior vary according to race or gender. For example, homosexual activity is the primary route of transmission of the AIDS virus for white males. However, although IV drug abuse is the primary route of transmission for black and Hispanic males, homosexual activity is an almost equivalent route of transmission. For black, white, and Hispanic females, IV drug use is the primary route of transmission and sexual activity with a male at risk (IVDU or bisexual male) at this time is a secondary transmission route. This pattern of risk may change as the epidemic continues, since more women may become infected with the AIDS virus through sexual activity with men at risk. Among males, whites account for 47 percent of the cases, followed by blacks (29 percent) and Hispanics (24 percent); among females, blacks account for 51 percent of the cases, followed by Hispanics (32 percent) and whites (16 percent). For adult cases, the ratio of men to women diagnosed with AIDS is about 7.8 cases to 1. However, the ratio of male IVDUs, including those who also engaged in homosexual activity, to female IVDUs diagnosed with AIDS is about 4.6 cases to 1. Also, IVDUs account for about 37 percent of the adult AIDS cases.

In April 1988, the New York City Department of Health reported that for the first 3 months of 1988, IVDUs accounted for 386 new AIDS cases, and homosexual and bisexual men accounted for 385 new cases. This was the first quarterly period where the number of newly reported AIDS cases among IVDUs equaled or surpassed the number reported among homosexual and bisexual men (S. Joseph 1988).

Of the 273 pediatric cases reported to the New York City Department of Health as of February 1988, approximately 73 percent were known to have parents, one or both of whom were IVDUS, and 4 percent (10) had mothers who were former sexual partners of IVDUs. An analysis of the ethnicity of 257 mothers of the pediatric cases showed that 60 percent were black, 32 percent were Hispanic, and 8 percent were white. Of the 9,047 babies born in New York City during a 4-week period in November and December of 1987, 148 (1.64 percent) tested positive for the presence of human immunodeficiency virus (HIV) antibodies, indicating that their mothers were infected. This is an infection rate of 1 out of every 61 women who gave birth during this period in New York City. Also, about 30 percent to 50 percent of these babies were probably infected (New York State Department of Health 1988). The remaining HIV-positive babies had possibly acquired antibodies from their mothers and were not themselves infected.

On any given day there are 10 children, hospitalized with HIV infection, who are ready for discharge and subsequent placement. The Foster Care Division of the New York City Human Resources Administration has recruited foster parents for children diagnosed with HIV infection, AIDS, or AIDS-related complex (ARC). Foster parents are paid an Exceptional Reimbursement Rate ($1,134 per month) plus money for diapers and clothing. The children's medical expenses are paid through Medicaid (Mayberry, personal communication, 1988).

As of February 1988, approximately 56 percent of the adult AIDS cases and 75 percent of the pediatric cases reported in New York City were known to have died. In 1986, although AIDS ranked fifth as a cause of death for all age groups in New York City, it was the major cause of death for adults between the ages of 25 and 44 (table 2). For the first time, in October of 1987, the number of deaths among intravenous drug abusers with AIDS surpassed the number of AIDS deaths among homosexual and bisexual men.

TABLE 2. *Number and percent of deaths in 1986 caused by AIDS in specific age groups by sex*

Age Group	Male Deaths	Per-cent	Female Deaths	Per-cent	Rank of AIDS as Cause of Death
All Ages	2,265	5.7	385	1.1	5
1 to 14	19	6.9	22	9.6	5
15 to 24	63	6.2	22	6.6	4
25 to 34	743	27.6	186	18.5	1
35 to 44	937	27.1	107	8.7	1
45 to 64	474	5.0	30	0.5	5

SOURCE: New York City Department of Health, Bureau of Health Statistics and Analysis (1986).

The above cases were classified as AIDS cases using the definition of the Centers for Disease Control in Atlanta. However, a study released by the New York City Department of Health, the New York State Division of Substance Abuse Services (DSAS), and Narcotic and Drug Research, Inc., used an expanded definition of AIDS-related deaths to include conditions associated with the presence of the AIDS virus: endocarditis, tuberculosis, oral thrush, and unusual pneumonias. Therefore, an additional 2,520 deaths of IVDUs were reclassified as AIDS-related for the period 1982 through 1986. Consequently, IVDUs accounted for 53 percent of the AIDS-related deaths and were considered the primary group at risk for HIV infection. Homosexual and bisexual men accounted for 38 percent of the deaths; an additional 4 percent were IVDUs who admitted to homosexual activity. About 5 percent of the deaths were in other risk categories, e.g., pediatric cases, hemophiliacs, and sexual partners of drug abusers (Stoneburner et al. 1987).

Preliminary reports generated by DSAS indicated that there was a large increase in the number of first-reported AIDS cases and the number of reported AIDS deaths in methadone maintenance programs from 1985 to 1987. Also, preliminary reports from an ongoing study at Beth Israel Medical Center by Dr. Beverly Richman have shown that AIDS is the number one cause of death, followed by alcoholism, in their methadone maintenance program of over 6,000 patients. Therefore, AIDS has emerged as the most serious growing health problem with high mortality rates within the methadone program.

Furthermore, studies estimating the HIV-antibody prevalence among patients entering methadone treatment vary from about 21 percent in suburban clinics in the Long Island/Queens area to about 60 percent in clinics located in inner-city neighborhoods of the Bronx, Brooklyn, and Manhattan (Magura, personal communication, 1987; Brown, personal communication, 1987). Of the estimated 258,000 narcotics addicts in New York State, approximately 200,000 reside in New York City. About 36,000 of the estimated number of opiate addicts in New York State are in methadone treatment, and another 1,900 are in drug-free programs. Based on the studies of HIV prevalence among addicts entering methadone programs, it is estimated that perhaps 50 percent to 60 percent of the opiate-addicted population in New York City (between 100,000 and 120,000 individuals) are HIV seropositive (Fenlon, personal communication, 1988; Des Jarlais, personal communication, 1988).

Increases in the number of newly reported tuberculosis and syphilis cases in New York City may be related to poverty, homelessness, and the presence of underlying HIV infection associated with IV drug abuse. Since 1979, the number of newly reported cases of tuberculosis has increased, especially among poor 25- to 44-year-old black males. The rate of newly reported tuberculosis cases has increased

215

from 22.7 cases per 100,000 persons in 1982 to 32.8 cases per 100,000 in 1987 (New York State Department of Health 1988). In 1985 and 1986, the health districts covering Central Harlem and the Lower East Side reported the highest rates of tuberculosis for health districts in the city (New York City Department of Health 1988b). Further, about 5 percent of the AIDS cases were diagnosed with tuberculosis, and the two diseases were diagnosed closely in time. These factors suggest that the resurgence of tuberculosis may be caused by the presence of HIV infection (City Health Information 1988).

The rate of primary and secondary syphilis increased from 29.2 cases per 100,000 persons in 1986 to 62.4 cases per 100,000 persons in 1987, while the rate of latent syphilis increased from 27.7 cases per 100,000 persons in 1986 to 48.1 cases per 100,000 persons in 1987 (New York State Department of Health 1988). Similarities in the geographical locations and demographics of age and sex of newly reported cases of AIDS and syphilis among IVDUs, including those who inject heroin and/or cocaine, and crack users, may suggest a possible relationship in the transmission of these diseases through the use of shared needles and sexual promiscuity. Studies completed in 1988 in New York City and San Francisco showed that cocaine IVDUs may be at higher risk than heroin IVDUs for transmitting and contracting the AIDS virus. Cocaine IVDUs inject more frequently than heroin IVDUs and therefore may share a greater number of contaminated needles. In New York City a study of 18 addicts who used heroin exclusively and 32 addicts who used cocaine exclusively showed that 28 percent of heroin users and 66 percent of cocaine users tested positive for antibodies to the AIDS virus. A group of about 200 addicts who injected cocaine and heroin showed a rate of infection similar to the cocaine addicts (Friedman, personal communication, 1988).

Extent of Homelessness in New York City

Size of the Population. Over the past two decades, homelessness in New York City has reached epidemic proportions. It is difficult to estimate the number of homeless individuals in New York City. Estimates range from 35,000 to 90,000 persons, depending on the formula used for the calculation. In New York City, about 32,000 persons currently reside in emergency shelters and temporary housing provided by the Human Resources Administration of New York City and nonprofit groups including the Partnership for the Homeless, Inc. The Partnership is a consortium of religious organizations that offer food and shelter in churches and synagogues to homeless people

(Partnership for the Homeless 1988a). A survey of 45 of the Nation's largest cities conducted in 1988 by the Partnership revealed an estimated 5,000 homeless persons with AIDS (PWAs) in New York City and 20,000 nationwide. In 94 percent of the cities, the number of homeless PWAs is expected to increase in 1989. These figures do not include HIV-positive and asymptomatic persons (Partnership for the Homeless 1988b).

In addition to those assisted by various public, private, and religious agencies, there are homeless people living in the streets and in terminals, abandoned buildings, parks, and subways. In 1984, New York State authorities adopted the formula that the actual number of homeless may be 150 percent, in addition to those assisted in shelters and emergency housing, or a total of about 80,000 persons. However, the Partnership for the Homeless has arrived at a "guesstimate" of 52,000 to 58,000 individuals—men, women, and children—based on the assumption that the number is in the range of 60 to 80 percent in addition to those sheltered by various agencies. This more conservative calculation was used because of the many programs implemented during the past 4 years. Other groups have calculated the total number of homeless as 10 percent above the assisted level, but this has been rejected by the Partnership for the Homeless as too low an estimate when considering the number of people seeking help from the streets.

In addition to the "visible homeless," there are the "hidden homeless" --families and "couch people" who double or triple up with others in substandard and overcrowded conditions. It is estimated that there are about 120,000 to 150,000 families or between 400,000 and 500,000 men, women, and children in these circumstances (Partnership for the Homeless 1988). If even a small percentage of such people—as little as 5 percent—should be evicted by primary tenants or landlords of the apartments, the number of "visible" homeless would be substantially increased and overwhelm existing services and resources.

Within the past year, however, there has been a leveling off in the number of known homeless persons in public shelters and other shel-ter facilities operated by private not-for-profit groups. For example, 12,906 single adults were provided emergency shelter on January 26, 1988. This represents a 4.4 percent increase over the number housed (12,334) on January 26, 1987. However, in 1986 there was a 20 per-cent increase over 1985 figures for persons housed in shelters (Partnership for the Homeless 1988).

Description of the Population. Systematic demographic information on the homeless is not available. Nonetheless, in their study of shelter residents in the summer of 1987, Struening (1988) and Pittman (1988) found that in a weighted sample equivalent to 1,000 residents, 85 percent were men and 15 percent were women. About 75.7 percent were black non-Hispanic, 15.6 percent were Hispanic, 6.8 percent were white, and 1.9 percent were other. Furthermore, 43.3 percent did not complete high school, 35.9 percent finished high school, 16.5 percent attended college, 3.6 percent graduated from college, and 0.8 percent received graduate degrees. The mean age of the residents was about 35.2 years. Although the range of ages was between 18 and 70 or more years, about 72.4 percent of the sample were between the ages of 18 and 39. About 62 percent were never married, 5.2 percent were currently married, 3.5 percent were widowed, and 29 percent were separated or divorced.

IVDUs comprise a subset of the homeless population in New York City. DSAS estimates that 40 percent of the State's homeless are substance abusers. Of the 11,394 homeless substance abusers serviced by the DSAS Homeless Project, about 34 percent had a history of IV drug abuse.

An ethnographic exploratory study of 70 homeless street addicts was undertaken by DSAS' Street Research Unit in the fall of 1985. This unit monitors drug activity on the streets of New York City and consists of street workers who, as former drug abusers, are knowledgeable about street life and drug abuse. They are trained in ethnographic techniques of observation to obtain information.

The homeless addicts interviewed in this study used various accommodations for shelter. During the week preceding the interviews, homeless addicts may have experienced one or more different types of homelessness: 56 percent experienced "extreme" homelessness, sleeping on roofs and in subways, basements, abandoned buildings, and shelters; 47 percent stayed with relatives or friends. Many of the addicts used more than one type of housing during the week of the interview alternating between accommodations with friends or family and the streets; thus, the percentages add up to more than 100 percent. Since this study was undertaken during warm weather, only four (6 percent) of the addicts used the public shelter system. However, about 21 percent stated they intended to stay in public shelters during the winter, and 34 percent intended to sleep in public places, such as subways, instead of the shelters. In this study, the public shelter system was used by a minority of the homeless addicts (Frank et al. 1985).

Of the homeless addicts interviewed, 44 percent were black, 26 percent were Hispanic, and 24 percent were white. The majority, 76 percent, were male, and 82 percent were between the ages of 20 and 39. Most of the subjects used more than one drug within 3 days of the interview, with heroin, used by 74 percent of the subjects, and cocaine, used by 57 percent, as the two most popular drugs. The major reasons given for homelessness by the addicts were use of drugs, being put out by their families, homeless by choice, unable to hold on to money, unable to find a place to live, being cut off from public assistance, and unable to find work (Frank et al. 1985).

About half the homeless addicts in this study would consider entering residential treatment, while the remainder were not receptive to the idea. Some of the reasons given for their rejection of residential treatment included fear of constraints and restrictions in therapeutic communities, fear of having to reveal personal details of one's life in group situations, dislike of red tape, and unwillingness to give up their way of life (Frank et al. 1985).

An exploratory survey was conducted in February of 1988 among clients in drug treatment programs known to the Homeless Emergency Assistance Referral and Treatment (HEART) Project. Subjects were selected for interviews using the following three criteria: (1) homeless IVDU just prior to admission to the program; (2) resident in a contracted program for the homeless; and (3) client referred to treatment through the HEART Project. Thirty-eight clients identified as meeting the criteria agreed to be interviewed.

To determine the type of housing patterns experienced by the clients, questions were asked concerning their living accommodations 2 years prior to their contact with the HEART Project. The following four findings describe the type of homelessness and instability of housing accommodations experienced by the clients.

- Twenty-two clients lived undomiciled in the streets, terminals, abandoned buildings, parks, subways, or shelters. Of these 22, 15 alternated between the shelters and the streets.

- Seventeen individuals lived in single-room-occupancy hotels or furnished rooms.

- Twenty-one persons moved from apartment to apartment with no permanent address. For the purposes of this study they are known as the "hidden homeless" or "couch people."

- Twelve people resided with family or friends but were put out of the apartment because of their drug use.

Of the 38 persons interviewed, 26 had experienced more than one type of homelessness and were classified in two or more of the categories.

An exploratory study of 52 addicted inmates in the New York City Rikers Island jail facility applying for admission to drug treatment in Key Extended Entry Program (KEEP) was conducted during the summer of 1987. Within the past 5 years, 42 (81 percent) of the inmates had experienced several episodes of homelessness or unstable housing conditions in the shelters (31 persons), streets (10 persons), single-room-occupancy hotels (28 persons), and as couch persons moving from apartment to apartment with no primary stable tenancy (33 persons). At the time of their arrests in the summer of 1987, only 6 were residing in their own home, and 12 were staying with relatives. The remainder were living with friends (8), as couch people (9), in single-room-occupancy hotels (5), in shelters (2), and on the streets in abandoned buildings, basements, cars, etc. (10). Twenty-nine (56 percent) indicated that they would need help to obtain housing upon their release from jail (Joseph et al. 1988).

Urban Decay: A Factor in the Spread of IV Drug Abuse and AIDS

Dr. Roderick Wallace of the Department of Epidemiology and Social Medicine of the Albert Einstein College of Medicine studied the consequences of arson and the destruction of low-income housing in the South Bronx on the spread of IV drug abuse and AIDS in the Bronx (Wallace, in press). His study (Wallace, in press, 1988) showed that the population of areas where low-income housing was destroyed in the 1970s migrated to other neighborhoods. IVDUs were included in this migration, and, subsequently, new clusters of IV drug abuse were created. In the Bronx, HIV infection is spread principally through IV drug use. Therefore, Dr. Wallace contends that the continued destruction of affordable housing, if it is not replaced, will result in further population shifts with accompanying homelessness among the displaced population and new clusters of IV drug abuse with a high prevalence of HIV infection. Also, old neighborhood social networks and services were disrupted as a result of the population shifts. Effective future AIDS education and intervention programs will therefore require the structuring of new community networks and services.

This process in low-income areas--arson followed by the destruction of affordable low-income housing, homelessness, and subsequent population migration--is therefore not only an important element in the continuing spread of IV drug abuse and AIDS, but also hinders the delivery of effective educational, medical, and social services to control the AIDS epidemic within the targeted population. As the process of destruction of housing, homelessness, and migration continues, efforts to reach IVDUs will be made more difficult by the ever-increasing geographical areas that require intensive services (Wallace, personal communication, 1988; Wallace, in press, 1988).

Summary

Three conditions interact and affect the IVDU--the AIDS epidemic, homelessness, and the destruction of housing in low-income neighborhoods. The availability of drugs in low-income neighborhoods places segments of the population at risk for addiction, IV drug use, and HIV infection. Furthermore, the continued destruction of low-income affordable housing exacerbates the spread of diseases and contributes to the general state of homelessness that affects the most vulnerable segments of the poor black and Hispanic population. The studies presented in this section indicate that IVDUs in New York City are becoming the major group at risk for HIV infection and the group most responsible for its spread to their sexual partners and offspring. IVDUs are also an integral part of the homeless population living on the streets. The convergence of the medical and social problems presented in this section makes the delivery of services in traditional forms a difficult undertaking at best and further contributes to the ongoing pathological conditions.

RECENT POPULATION SURVEYS AND STUDIES

Several surveys and studies, some of which are exploratory in nature, have been done investigating drug-using behavior associated with AIDS and HIV infection among the homeless. Ethnographic street studies, surveys in the shelters, single-room-occupancy and low-priced hotels, interviews with inmates at the Rikers Island jail facility, and drug treatment programs that serve the homeless IVDUs have collected data. Homeless IVDUs were interviewed and observed under different environmental conditions--such as streets, drug abuse treatment programs, jails, and shelters—by different groups of workers, including former drug abusers employed as street workers, survey interviewers, physicians, and professional researchers.

AIDS Risk Behavior Related to Drug Abuse Among Residents of New York City

The New York State DSAS, in cooperation with the New York State Division of Alcoholism and Alcohol Abuse, contracted with Louis Harris and Associates, Inc., to conduct a telephone survey in 1986 (unpublished) on drug and alcohol behavior among New York State residents. A total of 6,368 respondents across the State 18 years of age and older participated in the survey. Included in the sample were a cross-section of 4,010 residents in households with telephones, with oversamples of residents of Hispanic origin (563), and residents between the ages of 18 and 24 years (501). There were additional samples of residents living in households without telephones (399), college students (483), and "transients" occupying shelters and low-priced hotels throughout the State (412).

For the purposes of this analysis, the 3,144 respondents who resided in New York City were classified by two types of living accommodations: (1) shelters and low-priced and single-room-occupancy hotels, and (2) "other" accommodations (e.g., apartments or houses). Table 3 presents the proportion of residents in the two types of living accommodations who admitted engaging in any lifetime needle use for the injection of nonprescription or illicit drugs. Although no question was asked about the recency of needle use, a question was asked about the recency of heroin use. Almost all needle users who specified what drug they used with a needle mentioned heroin (although some also used cocaine or amphetamine).

The main trend emerging from table 3 is that the proportion of persons involved in drug-using risk behaviors associated with AIDS—use of needles within their lifetime for injection of illegal drugs, use of heroin within the past 5 years and within the past 2 years—is about 15 times greater among the homeless and transients in shelters and low-income hotels than among persons in "other" more stable accommodations.

For residents in the two types of living accommodations outside of New York City, similar patterns of needle and heroin use were found with smaller percentages.

222

TABLE 3. *Percentages of New York City residents in different living accommodations with drug-using risk behaviors associated with AIDS*

Drug-Using Risk Behaviors Associated with AIDS	Living Accommodations	
	Shelters, Single-Room-Occupancy, and Low-Priced Hotels	Other Accommo-dations
Residents with Any Lifetime Needle Use	21%	1.5%
Residents with Any Lifetime Needle Use and Use of Heroin With-in Last 5 Years	12%	0.8%
Residents with Any Lifetime Needle Use and Use of Heroin With-in Last 2 Years	10%	0.6%
Base (N)	(270)	(2,874)

SOURCE: New York State Division of Substance Abuse Services
Statewide Household Survey (1986).

AIDS Risk Behavior Related to Drug Abuse Among the Homeless

The following four findings emerged from the survey of 38 HEART clients concerning the use of shared unsterilized needles and cookers in relation to the time they became aware of AIDS and the consequences of sharing needles.

- Clients were generally informed about AIDS and received their information from reliable sources. Only one person claimed he did not have information from a formal source. The most common sources of information for this group were treatment programs (29 percent), magazines or newspapers (25 percent), brochures issued by agencies about AIDS and risk behavior (24 percent),

TV (25 percent), radio (20 percent), family/friends/coworkers (18 percent), medical personnel (16 percent), or from other drug users (15 percent).

- Notwithstanding the information or the sources, 20 clients (52 percent) continued to share unsterilized needles and cookers and some continued to go to shooting galleries (rooms in abandoned buildings or apartments in tenements where addicts can rent needles and buy and inject drugs) for an average period of 2.7 years after hearing about AIDS, before they entered the HEART Program.

- Of those interviewed only 5 (13 percent) never shared needles or cookers or visited shooting galleries. Another 13 (34 percent) stopped sharing works before they heard about AIDS.

- Although all clients were aware of the dangers of sharing needles, none were aware of the dangers of sharing cookers.

This exploratory survey did not measure the frequency of use of unsterilized shared needles and cookers or the frequency of visits to shooting galleries for the period before and after the clients heard about AIDS. However, while homeless, the majority of the clients did continue sharing needles and cookers, behavior which could result in the individual's transmitting or contracting the virus. After place-ment in treatment by the HEART Project, however 10 clients (26 per-cent) voluntarily participated in AIDS education and testing programs in AIDS outreach centers.

The above findings are similar to those obtained in interviews of IVDUs and needle sellers by street researchers of the DSAS Street Research Unit in 1984 and 1987. In 1984, 89 street IVDUs and/or needle sellers regarded AIDS as a disease confined to homosexuals. In 1987, 53 percent of 108 IVDUs admitted sharing needles with at least one other person. Although many addicts preferred using sterilized needles, they would use any needle available if they were sick and needed drugs (Hopkins 1988; Hopkins, personal communication, 1988.).

However, as street IVDUs became aware of the AIDS epidemic, the demand for clean needles increased. Dealers began to offer "free needles" as an AIDS prevention measure with $25 purchases of heroin. Also to meet the demand for clean needles, some dealers would re-package old needles and sell them as "new" to unsuspecting addicts.

By 1987, there were indications that some street addicts were trying to protect themselves, since about 41 percent of the 108 addicts interviewed in 1987 attempted to clean their needles with boiling water, alcohol, or bleach. However, interviews in 1987 revealed that even with the fear of AIDS and knowledge about transmission, street addicts still used unsterilized needles if they were sick and clean needles were not available. Furthermore, if money was limited and the choice was between the purchase of needles or drugs, many of the street addicts bought the drugs (Des Jarlais and Hopkins 1985; Des Jarlais et al. 1985; Hopkins 1988).

Narcotic addicts (27 males and 25 females) applying for admittance to KEEP in the New York City Rikers Island jail facility were inter-viewed about their addiction, social, and criminal histories. During the week prior to their arrest, the 52 inmates claimed to have spent about $7,700 per day on drugs—this expense was mostly for heroin and cocaine—which were administered by injection; about 85 percent admitted injecting cocaine within a 2-month period of their arrest. They averaged about 21 arrests per individual during the course of their addictions (females, 28 arrests vs males, 14.4 arrests). Only 6 were employed at the time of their arrests, 10 received public assis-tance, and 36 had no legal means of support (Joseph et al. 1988).

When 23 males were questioned about their use of shared, unsterilized needles, 18 indicated they had shared unsterilized needles within 2 years of their current arrests. The inmates were aware that shared, unsterilized needles are transmission routes for the AIDS virus, and there were indications that some individuals avoided sharing needles to avoid contracting AIDS. Three individuals stopped sharing needles in 1986, two in 1985, and two in 1984 (Joseph et al. 1988).

None of the males interviewed were aware that cookers could be a transmission route for the AIDS virus. Of the 22 males interviewed about their use of shared cookers, 20 indicated they had shared cookers within the last 2 years: 19 in 1987, the year of their arrests, and 1 in 1986. Although the 25 female narcotic addicts who applied for admission to KEEP during the summer of 1987 were not systematically questioned about the use of shared, unsterilized needles and cookers, those who used heroin and cocaine admitted that IV Injection was the preferred route of administration. Furthermore, the women interviewed had long histories of IV drug abuse and were of childbearing age (Joseph et al. 1988).

Of the 52 inmates, 38 have a total of 81 children; 23 of the females have from 1 to 9 children and 15 of the males have from 1 to 7 children. Within this group of IVDUs, a high probability exists that HIV may be transmitted to the neonates (Joseph et al. 1988).

AIDS Risk Behavior Related to Drug Abuse Among Shelter Residents

Preliminary findings are available from the following two studies. In both surveys, a significant proportion of the homeless respondents admitted injecting heroin within the past 8 years, which places them at particular risk for contracting or transmitting the AIDS virus. Notwithstanding the high prevalence of IV narcotics addiction within the shelter system, onsite methadone programs and detoxification services are currently not available for a number of administrative reasons. Because most programs to treat addicts are filled to capacity in New York City, it is difficult to place many homeless IV narcotic addicts in treatment immediately.

The first survey was conducted in the summer of 1987 by Dr. Elmer Struening and John Pittman of the New York State Psychiatric Institute. A preliminary analysis of the Struening-Pittman survey of a weighted sample equivalent to 1,000 residents in the 26 New York City-operated shelters showed that 10.4 percent were hospitalized at least once for a drug problem, and 10.7 percent had used opiates within the 6-month period prior to the interview. Also, 18 percent admitted using heroin more than 50 times during their lives, 36 percent admitted using cocaine more than 60 times, and 18 percent admitted using crack over 70 times. This group included current daily abusers of heroin, cocaine, and crack. The three drugs present a serious risk of transmitting and contracting AIDS because of the use of shared contaminated needles by heroin and cocaine IVDUs and possible sexual promiscuity as a result of smoking crack (Struening and Pittman, 1988; Struening, personal communication, 1988; Pittman, personal communication, 1988). This group included current daily abusers of heroin. About 11 percent admitted injecting drugs since 1980.

Preliminary findings of an ongoing survey conducted by Dr. Ernest Drucker of the Department of Epidemiology and Social Medicine of the Montefiore Medical Center show that between 35 percent and 40 percent of 115 recent admissions to the Franklin Men's Shelter in the Bronx admit to current episodes of IV heroin use. Abuse of cocaine and crack are also major problems within this shelter population (Drucker, personal communication, 1988).

HIV Infection in the Shelters

The number of homeless AIDS or ARC patients is unknown, since many of these individuals try to conceal their illness. Although patients with AIDS or ARC are not officially discharged from hospitals to shelters, PWAs who are evicted from their apartments or rooms may seek living accommodations within the shelter system. Also, another group of homeless individuals with AIDS or ARC may have developed these conditions without episodes of hospitalization and therefore are part of an unofficial or "hidden" infected population.

If they are forced to use shelters, people with AIDS, ARC, or HIV infection conceal their conditions. Many fear they will be intimidated and threatened with physical violence if their condition becomes known to other shelter residents. If discovered by physicians or social workers within the shelter system, AIDS patients are referred to proper medical facilities and moved to other quarters (Drucker, personal communication, 1988; McAdam, personal communication, 1988).

The majority of the shelter respondents participating in the survey conducted by Struening (1988) and Pittman (1988) were concerned about the consequences of the AIDS epidemic. Table 4 summarizes their responses to specific questions about AIDS. The majority perceived AIDS as a problem in the shelters. Also, while the majority (55 percent) were worried about getting AIDS, only about one-third (31 percent) indicated they had a good or fair chance of contracting the disease.

The Department of Community Medicine of St. Vincent's Hospital administers a medical program servicing the residents of the Keener Men's Shelter on Ward's Island in New York City. Three physicians and three nurses are assigned to this project, which offers physical examinations and medical care for acute conditions, trauma, and chronic conditions (such as tuberculosis) in a medical unit housed within the shelter. The shelter is run by the Volunteers of America under contract to the New York City Human Resources Administration. With a capacity of 816 beds, the shelter services about 1,200 men per month (Woods, personal communication, 1988). It is estimated that about 10 percent of the shelter residents request medical

TABLE 4. *Perception of shelter residents regarding AIDS epidemic (sample weighted to 1,000 residents)*

Question	Positive Response (Percent)
(1)　Is AIDS a big problem in the shelters?	59.2
(2)　Do you know anyone who has AIDS?	15.3
(3)　Do you worry about getting AIDS?	54.8
(4)　What are your chances of getting AIDS?	
good	8.6
fair	22.8
poor	23.1
none	33.5
other and don't know	12.0

attention from the St. Vincent's medical unit (McAdam, personal communication, 1988).

In August of 1986, Dr. John McAdam, one of the physicians assigned to the Keener Men's Shelter, started an informal exploratory study of possible HIV infection among men who were in known risk groups: IVDUs, men engaging in homosexual activity, sexual partners at risk, and men who received blood transfusions. Eventually two other physicians were enlisted to assist in the project. The physicians provided pretest and posttest counseling. From August of 1986 to March of 1988, 35 residents agreed to be tested, with 30 of them tested between August of 1987 and March of 1988. One individual who was tested did not belong to a risk group but presented medical problems suggestive of underlying HIV infection.

The mean age of the residents tested was 33.1 years with an age range from 21 years to 46 years. About 80 percent of the residents tested were black, 14 percent were Hispanic, and 6 percent were white. Twenty-eight (80 percent) were found to be seropositive. Infection was found across all racial groups. Of the 23 IVDUs, 21 tested positive. Four residents (11 percent) had sufficient symptoms of ARC to qualify for AZT and were administered the medication while residing at the shelter. (One AZT patient died from an overdose of narcotics, and another was removed from the drug because of side effects.) Twenty-five patients (71 percent) reported for the results of the test. Of the 10 patients who did not report for their results, 9 were HIV positive (table 5) (McAdam, personal communication, 1988).

TABLE 5. *Prevalence of HIV seropositivity and followup status by risk group of male residents in a New York City shelter (n = 35)*

	Number Tested	Number Seropositive (%)	Number Reported for Results	Number on AZT (%)
IV Drug Use	20	20 (100)	12 (60)	3 (15)
Homosexual Activity	9	6 (66)	8 (89)	1 (11)
IV Drug Use and Homosexual Activity	3	1 (33)	2 (66)	0
Sex Partner at Risk	1	1 (100)	1 (100)	0
Blood Products	1	0	1 (100)	0
No-Risk Group	1	0	1 (100)	0
Total	35	28 (80)	25 (71)	4 (12)

The physicians and social worker reported that AIDS patients are not being discharged from hospitals into the Keener Shelter. Only one

AIDS case was reported of a homeless homosexual from another country; one individual who developed an advanced case of ARC was referred to Bailey House, a residence for PWAs. The problem in the Keener Shelter, therefore, is undetected HIV infection and residents with cases of ARC.

An AIDS prevention program has been developed in this shelter. The physicians and social worker inform residents about the use of clean needles to avoid contracting and transmitting HIV. Also, the Keener Shelter distributes condoms. IVDUs are referred to treatment. However, the lack of adequate treatment facilities in the community, especially methadone maintenance and detoxification services, has prevented many addicts from entering programs promptly.

Dr. McAdam and the other two physicians have demonstrated that voluntary testing and treatment with AZT is possible within a shelter setting. There has been an unusually high level of compliance by the 35 patients, as the majority reported for the results of the tests, and, for those eligible, the taking of prescribed AZT. This may be due to the personalized approach and counseling of the medical staff and the fact that all services—testing, physical examinations, counseling, and treatment with AZT—are available on site. Dr. McAdam estimates that about one-half of his patients in the Keener shelter have histories of IV drug abuse and that about 75 percent may be involved with crack.

Dr. Paul Perowsky of the Woodhull Hospital in Brooklyn, New York is the director of medical care for two shelters in Brooklyn: a men's shelter with a capacity to serve about 1,000 persons and a women's shelter with a capacity to serve about 150 persons. He estimates that about 300 to 400 residents in these shelters request medical care every month. Of this number, about 10 percent to 20 percent appear to be infected with HIV, and about one-half of those infected can be diagnosed as having AIDS in accordance with the criteria established by the CDC (Perowsky, personal communication, 1988).

The Franklin Avenue Men's Shelter in the Bronx was highlighted in an article in the *New York Times* on April 4, 1988 (Kolata 1988), concerning the plight of homeless PWAs living in the city shelters. Some of these people may not have received an official diagnosis of AIDS but have symptoms related to HIV infection. Although there are no surveys to determine the number of current PWAs in this particular shelter, Dr. Ernest Drucker of Montefiore Hospital estimates that about 40 percent of the 600 residents are IVDUs and another 5 percent are homosexual. He estimates that about 50 percent of each risk group are infected and about 20 percent show overt symptoms of AIDS or ARC (Drucker, personal communication, 1988).

In the winter of 1987 to 1988, Dr. Drucker studied the housing accommodations of 160 PWAs with histories of IV drug use who were admitted to six voluntary hospitals in New York City. About 10 percent were admitted to hospitals from shelters, another 10 percent were admitted homeless from the streets, and an additional 20 percent were either admitted from single-room-occupancy hotels or were living as "couch people" moving from apartment to apartment with no permanent residence. The remaining people had more stable living conditions (Drucker, personal communication, 1988).

Medical, Management, and Housing Problems of PWAs

The condition of homelessness among PWAs presents serious problems that affect the delivery of medical and social services, the patients' welfare, and the public health of the community at large. These problems were highlighted in a study conducted by Dr. Ramon A. Torres of the Department of Community Medicine of St. Vincent's Hospital in New York City of all 231 AIDS patients hospitalized at St. Vincent's Hospital from November 1981 to October 1985. Included in this sample were 36 AIDS patients (16 percent) identified as IVDUs. There were 30 patients (13 percent) considered homeless upon admission to the hospital. IVDUs constituted the majority—21 (70 percent)—of the homeless AIDS patients (Torres et al. 1987).

Management problems of homeless AIDS patients as compared to non-homeless AIDS patients are more difficult. These problems include higher rates of signing out of the hospital against medical advice, refusals to complete diagnostic tests and undergo treatment for opportunistic infection, broken outpatient appointments, longer hospital stays, lost prescriptions, and patients lost to medical followup.

Medical problems among the homeless AIDS patients include higher rates of tuberculosis and possibly pneumocystis carinii pneumonia (PCP) as compared to nonhomeless patients. Confirmation of PCP was less frequent among homeless patients since they were less willing to complete the diagnostic procedures (Torres, personal communication, 1988; Torres et al. 1987). Homeless AIDS patients may also exhibit the various forms of trauma, infestations, peripheral vascular disease, mental instability, and other conditions associated with some segments of the general homeless population (Brickner, personal communication, 1988; Brickner et al. 1986).

In the New York City Beth Israel Methadone Program, AIDS coordinators work with the patient and family as soon as HIV seropositivity is known or symptoms of infection are recognized. Plans for adequate housing are an integral part of counseling. If the patient does not have a family or a place to live and is ill, a referral is made to Bailey House, a residence for PWAs. However, because Bailey House has a limited capacity of 44 beds, many patients are referred to single-room-occupancy hotels and YMCAs upon hospital discharge or, if they are not ambulatory, to Bird S. Coler Hospital (Haig, personal communication, 1988).

Homeless PWAs released from prison are also referred to single-room-occupancy hotels or YMCAs. However, if referred to a Y, the patient must move every 28 days, in accordance with the Y's regulations prohibiting persons from establishing long-term residence. These types of accommodations are inadequate for many discharged from the hospitals and prisons. The patients usually cannot get nutritious food and are placed in environments where drugs are readily available. Patients may relapse to IV drug abuse and are subjected to further infection in inadequate housing. Unless patients are known to social workers or other service providers, they may neither receive services nor be able to comply with prescribed medical procedures (Springer, personal communication, 1988).

Followup of AIDS or ARC persons known to the Association for Drug Abuse Prevention and Treatment (ADAPT) has shown that the majority released from jails die within 3 or 4 months. ADAPT workers report that PWAs feel isolated in furnished rooms and in some instances have been found ill and alone in their rooms for several days. When this occurs, ADAPT workers have had to call for medical help or escort the patient to a hospital (Serrano, personal communication, 1988).

Summary

Surveys and exploratory studies focused on drug-related risk behavior associated with AIDS indicate that as housing accommodations become more unstable, the proportion of residents admitting to IV heroin use or any lifetime use of needles for injecting illicit drugs increases significantly. Homeless addicts interviewed on the streets, in jails, or in treatment programs were aware of the danger of transmitting or contracting AIDS through use of shared needles. Although attempts were made, these addicts were unable to translate knowledge into consistent risk-free behavior. Physicians affiliated with shelters are now seeing evidence of HIV infection, ARC, and AIDS among the homeless residents who are IVDUs and/or homosexuals. Also, based on the cited studies, homeless AIDS patients have greater rates of tuberculosis than nonhomeless patients, present serious medical management problems, and may not be able to comply with prescribed procedures.

EXISTING AND NEEDED PROGRAMS

Housing for Homeless AIDS Patients

The plight of homeless PWAs has received extensive media coverage. Attempts over the past 2 years to establish residential and service centers for PWAs have generated a considerable amount of community resistance in New Jersey, Queens, and Manhattan. In addition to community approval and site selection, funding and program issues have to be resolved. Notwithstanding these obstacles, The AIDS Resource Center, Inc., a private nonprofit organization in New York City, currently has succeeded in establishing two model housing programs for homeless PWAs: the Scatter Site Apartment Program and the Bailey House Congregate Residence. Because of limited facilities, the AIDS Resource Center is able to house about one out of six homeless PWAs who are referred for help. Each program is an example of support housing with three common features:

(1)   a permanent affordable home that can be used until more intensive medical care is required;

(2)   a wide range of social, medical, and recreational services, either within the residence or in the community (e.g., individual and group counseling, recreational activities, information about and referrals to medical facilities, availability of spiritual care); and

(3)   home care services (Fisher 1988).

The Scatter Site Apartment Program is currently in operation with 15 units and has a capacity to serve 17 PWAs or 23 persons if other family members, such as spouses and children, are included. This program offers independent apartment living in various neighborhoods. The program protects confidentiality since only the landlord is aware of the tenant's condition and the location of the apartment.

233

Therefore, there is no organized community opposition. The apartments have a private kitchen, toilet, and bathing facilities. Residents can prepare their own meals and, if necessary, apply for and receive home care services. PWAs from all risk groups are accepted into this program (Fisher 1988; Fisher, personal communication, 1988).

Bailey House, established in December of 1986, is a converted hotel in Greenwich Village with a capacity for housing 44 single adults. Unlike the Scatter Site Apartment Program, confidentiality about the resident's AIDS diagnosis is not an issue since residents must have AIDS to qualify for admission, and the residence is designated as serving this particular group. The program has been accepted by the residents of the neighborhood.

All rooms have private toilet and bathing facilities. Three nutritious meals are served daily in a central dining area. In addition to the communal dining facility, each floor has areas for socialization. Staff includes a full-time nurse, personal care assistants to help with room cleaning, shopping, and other assistance that the resident may require. In addition, there are social workers who assist patients with personal problems. Help with substance abuse is available. All former heroin addicts are served by community methadone programs. If the patient is too ill to report for medication, the program will deliver methadone to the patient at Bailey House. Residents can choose to use a variety of community outpatient or inpatient medical services. Also, the Visiting Nurse Service provides ongoing care for persons too ill to go to clinics and may assign personal health aides to individual residents (Haugh, personal communication, 1988; Fisher 1988).

The program accepts PWAs from all risk groups. At present, about half are homosexual or bisexual males, and the rest are former IV heroin addicts. Despite the residents' varied backgrounds, congregate living has encouraged positive interaction, with residents helping each other and visiting those who are hospitalized. The control of episodes of acute pain, however, is reported to be a major problem for many AIDS patients in the residence. Prescribed medication for effective relief of pain and depression is indicated, since some residents may resort to the use of nonprescribed substances to obtain relief (Haugh, personal communication, 1988).

Within the past year, hospitals and methadone programs have referred homeless patients to Bailey House to address the posthospitalization housing needs of homeless AIDS patients. As a result of increased social services and stable housing conditions, homeless AIDS patients who entered were better able to comply with medical followup (Torres, personal communication, 1988).

Daytop Village, a drug-free therapeutic community, has developed an extensive AIDS program, which offers education to staff and residents. Drug abusers with AIDS can enter Daytop and are placed in a special program that has been developed by the staff in consultation with physicians. Most AIDS patients who participate in this program are homeless. Residents with AIDS remain in Daytop when asymptomatic or when the illness is stabilized, are hospitalized during periods of acute illness, and return to Daytop after their discharge from the hospital. While in Daytop, other residents are assigned to assist AIDS patients. Physicians knowledgeable about AIDS and drug abuse treat and monitor the residents with AIDS. Also, AIDS patients afflicted with pain are prescribed analgesics while living in the therapeutic community. The program admits only a limited number of AIDS patients, since many patients might have a detrimental impact on the program for the other residents. However, the procedures developed at Daytop can be used as a model for the treatment of AIDS patients within the setting of a therapeutic community (Sorrell, personal communication, 1988).

As of February 28, 1988, the Division of AIDS Services of the New York City Human Resources Administration served about 1,400 (22 percent) of the 6,500 persons diagnosed as having AIDS in the city by providing couseling, home care, and nursing and family support services. Also, the agency meets the specific housing needs of 21 patients in scatter-site housing, 41 patients in Bailey House, 129 patients in single-room-occupancy hotels, and 596 patients in apartments (Triscari, personal communication, 1988).

In 1982, DSAS established a residence known as the Short Stay Program as part of the drug treatment services offered by the Lower East Service Center in Manhattan for marginal methadone patients with multiple drug abuse problems, who were homeless. This program is not designed for AIDS patients, but is a model program for homeless patients who may be injecting drugs. Residents are referred from methadone clinics and are maintained on methadone for their course of treatment, which usually lasts from 3 to 6 months. During this period, patients' problems and housing needs are addressed and, when ready, the resident is transferred back to the referring program. Within the next year, homeless addicts eligible for methadone treatment will be referred to the program.

Efforts to Expand Treatment Intake

The Homeless Project. The Homeless Project organized by the New York State DSAS consists of two components—The HEART Project and the Shelter Referral Project. The HEART Project was conceived in May of 1985 by Julio Martinez, the director of DSAS, in response to Governor Cuomo's mandate "to develop programs to address the plight of the homeless." This program was designed to serve homeless substance abusers. Mobile vans are used as intake and referral offices in neighborhoods where addicts congregate. Homeless addicts are interviewed about their backgrounds: drug, treatment, and criminal histories; social and demographic data; and medical and psychiatric histories. Assessments for the type of help that is needed and appropriate referrals for placement in detoxification and/or residential facilities are then completed.

The initial steps for the HEART Project were to develop a residential drug-free treatment modality for homeless drug abusers and to fund treatment programs to provide appropriate services. Vans staffed with DSAS personnel experienced in engaging active substance abusers were located in places where addicts congregate. Input about locations for the vans was obtained from the DSAS Street Research Unit, community-based organizations, and volunteer groups. Linkages were developed with offices of New York City's Borough Presidents, and additional data were gathered through the Agency's toll-free information telephone line.

Referrals were obtained from shelters, since DSAS participates in an interagency effort with the New York State Office of Mental Health and the New York State Division of Alcoholism and Alcohol Abuse to provide outreach services to homeless substance abusers in New York City's Municipal Shelter System. Teams of workers from the three agencies are sent to shelters to interview residents. Clients are interviewed about their drug abuse histories and need for treatment. Referrals to treatment programs are made from the shelters, and residents are placed if an opening is available.

By April 15, 1988, 11,394 homeless substance abusers were served by the Homeless Project. However, 1,814 returned on two or more occasions for services. Therefore, the number of total client contacts was 13,208. IV substance abusers accounted for 34 percent of those served.

Tables 6, 7, and 8 summarize the interviews for the Homeless Project. Approximately 43 percent of the total client contacts were referred to programs; 57 percent were not referred for various reasons. Less than 1 percent of the contacts refused assistance. There were no significant differences in the outcomes for those interviewed by the HEART Project or the Shelter Referral Project. Practically all clients interviewed in the Homeless Project accepted some type of help for their drug abuse problems.

TABLE 6. *Number of clients interviewed in homeless projects*

Category	HEART Project	Shelter Project	Total
New Clients Seen	6,431 (100%)	4,963 (100%)	11,394 (100%)
Returnees	889 (14%)	925 (19%)	1,814 (16%)
Total Contacts	7,320 (100%)	5,888 (100%)	13,208 (100%)
Referred to Rx	3,121 (43%)	2,564 (44%)	5,685 (43%)
Not Referred	4,199 (57%)	3,324 (56%)	7,523 (57%)

Of the 5,685 persons referred to treatment programs, 52 percent were referred to residential drug-free programs contracted by the HEART Project, and 17 percent were referred to other residential drug-free programs. The others were referred to detoxification facilities (21 percent), social service agencies (9 percent), and other types of treatment (1 percent). Of the 7,523 not referred to specific programs, 84 percent were placed on waiting lists, with an additional 8 percent being placed on waiting lists and referred to shelters, since there were no openings in the treatment programs. About 7 percent received counseling on the van for their drug problems. As of March 1988, 563 homeless clients were in specifically funded drug-free residential programs contracted by the HEART Project. Of this number, 89 (16 percent) were IVDUs (Fenlon, personal communication, 1988).

TABLE 7. *Type of referrals made by the homeless projects*

Type of Referral	HEART Project	Shelter Project	Total
HEART Residential Drug-Free Program	1,936 (62%)	992 (39%)	2,928 (52%)
Other Residential Drug-Free Program	366 (12%)	595 (23%)	961 (17%)
Detoxification	536 (17%)	672 (26%)	1,208 (21%)
Ambulatory			
Drug-Free Program	3 (*)	19 (*)	22 (*)
Methadone Program	5 (*)	30 (1%)	35 (*)
Alcohol	2 (*)	2 (*)	19 (*)
Other	17 (*)	2 (*)	19 (*)
Social Service Referrals	256 (8%)	234 (9%)	490 (9%)
Total	3,121 (100%)	2,564 (100%)	5,685 (100%)

KEY: (*) = less than 1 percent.

Key Extended Entry Program (KEEP). KEEP was created in 1986 by Mr. Charles Laporte, Director of the New York State DSAS Bureau of Chemotherapy Services (BCS) and his staff to help meet the following objectives:

(1) to facilitate the entry of untreated heroin addicts into long-term treatment for their drug addiction;

(2) to curtail the AIDS epidemic among IVDUs by offering treatment for drug abuse and education about AIDS;

(3) to reduce criminal activity related to IV drug abuse; and

(4) to help relieve overcrowded jail conditions.

238

TABLE 8. *Status of clients not referred to treatment*

Status	HEART	Shelter	Total
Clients Placed on Waiting List	3,514 (84%)	2,802 (84%)	6,316 (84%)
Clients Placed on Waiting List and Referred to Shelters	624 (18%)	0	624 (8%)
Clients Who Received Information and Counseling	32 (*)	486 (14%)	500 (7%)
Refused Referral	29 (*)	54 (2%)	83 (1%)
Total Not Referred to Programs	4,199 (100%)	3,324 (100%)	7,523 (100%)

KEY: (*) = less than 1 percent.

The program was developed in the New York City Department of Correctional Services (DOCS) detoxification facilities on Rikers Island and in community-based methadone programs. Patients are recruited for KEEP from the following sources: (1) walk-in applicants from the streets who come to the programs in search of treatment; (2) referrals from AIDS outreach units; (3) methadone maintenance program waiting lists; and (4) inmates incarcerated at the Rikers Island jail facility.

Persons who enter KEEP are initially placed on a detoxification schedule of up to 180 days. During this 6-month period, patients are maintained on doses of methadone sufficient to curtail heroin abuse and are evaluated for placement in appropriate long-term treatment. The decision about placement in long-term treatment is based on the results of medical examinations, the duration of the patient's addiction, the patient's preferences, and an evaluation of the patient's behavior, needs, and adjustment during a 1½- to 6-month period. The patient may be accepted into methadone maintenance treatment or referred to an alternative program such as a therapeutic community, methadone-to-abstinence program, or drug-free counseling. If a drug-free program is selected, the patient completes the detoxification process by reducing the dose of methadone to zero in a controlled series of steps. Twelve community-based methadone programs are currently participating in this program.

KEEP at the Rikers Island correctional facility was organized from March through August of 1987 by staff members of DSAS/BCS in conjunction with the DOCS and the Montefiore-Rikers Island health facility. The staff of BCS designed the program, planned its implementation, and administered the program for the first 2 months of operation. Subsequently, appropriate staff were hired by Montefiore-Rikers Island health services to operate the program in conjunction with DOCS. However, the staff of BCS continues to provide technical assistance. Inmates voluntarily elect to enter the program from the detoxification wards operated by the Montefiore Medical Center on Rikers Island in three facilities: the correctional institution for women (presentenced and sentenced females), the correctional institution for men (sentenced men) and the Anna M. Kross Center (presentenced men).

KEEP at Rikers Island is a major innovation. For the first time in a prison system, opiate-addicted inmates eligible to enter community-based treatment are maintained on 30 mg to 40 mg of methadone a day until their release. While incarcerated, inmates are educated about AIDS risk behavior associated with transmitting and contracting the virus and ways to prevent transmission. Within 24 hours of their release, they are administered a dose of methadone and referred to a community KEEP methadone program for continued treatment and evaluation. The program has proven to be effective in reducing tensions and discipline problems within the treated population of the jail.

Of the first 1,146 admissions discharged to the community-based methadone programs, 786 (69 percent) reported for and were accepted into treatment. Males had a higher reporting rate than females (73 percent vs 63 percent). There are indications that female prostitution may be a factor in the females' lower reporting rate (Joseph et al. 1988).

KEEP in the city jails is an example of frontline medicine. The program provides medical services onsite where potential patients, the majority of whom were homeless or in unstable living accommodations, may be recruited for treatment. By establishing KEEP, the traditional intake process has been modified to accommodate populations who are either intimidated by the intake process or who have been unable to organize their lives to apply for treatment.

AIDS Outreach and Prevention Programs. The AIDS Outreach and Prevention program (AOP) operates in the boroughs of Manhattan, Brooklyn, the Bronx, and Queens from various sites in selected neighborhoods where there is a high incidence of IV drug abuse. Outreach workers who are former drug abusers canvass the neighborhood locating drug abusers to educate them about AIDS, risk reduction behavior, and treatment. Referrals are made to various community services, including drug treatment programs. Drug abusers are also informed about HIV-antibody testing. If they agree to be tested, they are brought to a test site operated by the New York State Department of Health. The client also receives pre- and posttest counseling at the Department of Health office.

A mobile van is used to distribute AIDS information to the general community and to make contact with nonaddicted relatives and friends of drug addicts. Family members and friends are encouraged to refer addicted relatives and friends to the program. The program also distributes an AIDS photonovel about risk behavior and ways to avoid transmitting or contracting the virus (Mauge, personal communication, 1988). The photonovel uses still photos to depict a story about a young substance abuser and his sexual partner and their concerns about AIDS risk behavior. Actors depict situations. Dialog about AIDS and risk behavior is presented in comicbook-style balloons. English and Spanish photonovels are being distributed in New York City.

AIDS MOBILE OUTREACH PROJECT

The AIDS Mobile Outreach Project will be in operation in 1989 and will focus on particular neighborhoods in New York City and Albany with a high incidence of AIDS, high mortality rates related to AIDS, and a high incidence of children born with HIV antibodies. The distinguishing feature of this program will be the use of professional social workers and substance abuse counselors to establish comprehensive education, counseling, and referral services in AIDS-related matters to substance abusers who reside, or who may be homeless, in the area. Vans will be deployed to the targeted neighborhoods. Substance abusers will be counseled and educated about AIDS, and the behavior modification techniques necessary to reduce transmitting and contracting the virus will be discussed. Videotapes instructing substance abusers about AIDS and risk-reduction behavior will be shown. Also, risk-reduction materials will be distributed including literature (photonovels, pamphlets), condoms, and bleach. Referrals will be made to appropriate social services, treatment programs, and HIV testing sites (Wender, personal communication, 1988).

COMMUNITY AIDS PREVENTION OUTREACH DEMONSTRATION PROJECT

Additional outreach programs are being implemented that will involve distributing condoms and bleach for sterilizing needles. Also, formal self-help groups composed of individuals from different risk groups (e.g., prostitutes, female IVDUs, male heterosexual IVDUs, and female sex partners of male IVDUs) will be created to reduce risk behavior. These groups will be led by experienced professional group leaders.

Street-level self-help groups are organized by trained ex-addict facilitators. The groups are composed of IVDUs and others who may be part of their friendship circles and meet where addicts congregate. Outreach workers attempt to develop impromptu discussions about AIDS, testing, and risk behavior reduction. The major purpose of these groups is the development of new behavioral norms, rituals, and practices by IVDUs to reduce risk behavior, both individually and within the group. In addition to providing information, the groups offer a place to express beliefs and fears about AIDS, testing, death, sexual practices, and rejection. It is also hoped that the participants will be empowered to change their behavior, impart their knowledge to other IVDUs, and promote new norms and practices that would reduce risk behavior among extended groups of IVDUs. In addition to discussions, referrals are made to drug treatment programs and other types of services (Friedman, personal communication, 1988). A recently funded AIDS outreach and demonstration project will focus on the Harlem community, engaging both IVDUs and their sexual partners in counseling efforts to reduce risk behaviors (Deren, personal communication, 1988). ADAPT participates in these projects, helping to organize street-level groups, educate addicts, and refer them to treatment and services.

The Association for Drug Abuse Prevention and Treatment (ADAPT). ADAPT was originally organized in the late 1970s to merge the various philosophies and approaches for drug treatment. In

242

response to the AIDS epidemic, the organization was reconstituted in 1986 under the leadership of Yolanda Serrano to educate drug abusers about AIDS, to advocate programs for drug abusers to curtail the epidemic, to refer IVDUs to treatment, and to develop programs to meet those objectives. The organization consists of former substance abusers, drug treatment personnel, physicians, patients enrolled in drug treatment, researchers, and other interested parties.

ADAPT has organized a program to assist hospitalized AIDS and ARC patients in the New York City jails. Patients are helped with housing and social service referrals upon their release from jail, since many of the patients have been abandoned by families and friends. Also, for those who remain in the institution, assistance is provided for legal and family matters, grievances about conditions, and AIDS education and treatment opportunities.

Outreach efforts to educate and offer services to street addicts is an integral part of ADAPT's program. Teams of ADAPT members have gone into communities, shooting galleries, shelters, and abandoned buildings where homeless drug abusers congregate to educate them about safe sex practices, to instruct addicts how to clean needles with bleach, and to distribute small packages containing a vial of bleach, a vial of water, cotton, and a condom. ADAPT currently backs the establishment of a needle exchange program in New York City and is participating in research, education, and service outreach programs aimed at hard-core street addicts who do not avail themselves of services offered by formal institutions (Serrano, personal communication, 1988).

Homeless Health Initiative. To serve homeless people, including approximately 4,000 families in shelters and hotels, New York City established the Homeless Health Initiative. The program is intended to address unmet needs within this population. Standards and policies that affect the population positively were developed. Monitoring relevant health and environmental outcomes and interacting with other agencies to develop programs are essential project components. Programs serve families and individuals in shelters and hotels and focus on alcohol and drug abuse, mental illness, general health assessment, health education, referrals to community facilities, adverse environmental conditions in shelters and hotels, services for pregnant women and neonates, child abuse, and infant mortality. When applicable, referrals are made to community agencies and programs. Onsite services staffed by health workers and public health nurses have also been developed.

THE NEED FOR TREATMENT

Treatment for the IVDU

The demand for treatment of IVDUs has resulted in a 105 percent
utilization of the treatment capacity of funded methadone programs in
New York State. In March 1988, 34,568 patients were enrolled in
State-funded and private methadone maintenance programs in New
York State, and 1,088 were enrolled in methadone-to-abstinence programs (Management Information System 1988). An additional 975
narcotics addicts were on waiting lists to enter methadone programs
in New York State (Bureau of Chemotherapy Services 1988). To
address the urgent demand for treatment and the problem of AIDS,
Governor Cuomo directed the New York State DSAS to add 5,000
additional methadone treatment slots in 1988.

In the early 1970s, there were waiting periods of up to 24 months to
enter methadone treatment. Clinics known as holding units were
opened to provide immediate treatment to addicts on waiting lists.
These clinics offered minimal services. Their purpose was to expand
treatment intake as quickly as possible for those addicts who applied
and were waiting for admission. When placements opened in regular
methadone clinics, patients were transferred for continued treatment.
A similar model, known as the Interim Clinic, was created in 1986 by
Beth Israel Medical Center as an AIDS prevention measure, to bring
persons on waiting lists into treatment as quickly as possible. The
KEEP community programs affiliated with 12 methadone programs are
also based on the holding clinic model. They accept addicts from
waiting lists for immediate treatment, evaluation, and eventual transfer to programs that offer long-term care and relevant services
(Bureau of Chemotherapy Services 1988).

In March 1988, State-funded, drug-free residential programs throughout New York State were utilized at 107 percent of funded capacity
and were treating about 4,808 clients. Of this number, 17 percent
were IVDUs. Of the 47,000 clients treated in State-funded programs,
72 percent were in treatment in New York City. The need for treatment is underscored by the fact that, in New York City, where the
AIDS epidemic is most prevalent, total treatment for drug abuse--
methadone maintenance, drug-free residential, drug-free day service,
drug-free day outpatient--is utilized at 104 percent of its funded
capacity (Fenlon, personal communication, 1988; Management Information System 1988).

Summary

A variety of projects have been developed by New York State and New York City agencies to meet the needs of homeless IVDUs and AIDS patients. By developing housing programs, outreach in the community, and expanded intake to allow a greater number of IV drug abusers to enter treatment, a comprehensive strategy could be created that would serve homeless AIDS patients and curb the spread of the epidemic. At present there is such a heavy demand for treatment and adequate housing for PWAs that drug treatment programs are over capacity, especially in areas with high levels of drug abuse and HIV infection.

SUMMARY AND CONCLUSIONS

This chapter summarizes the results of selected ongoing surveys, exploratory studies, interviews with physicians working with homeless IVDUs, and programs concerning AIDS and the homeless in New York City. Current statistical data from the New York City Department of Health show that IVDUs are now becoming the primary risk group for HIV infection in New York City. Interviews of homeless IV drug addicts incarcerated in Rikers Island jail facilities revealed that these addicts had long histories of involvement with the criminal justice system and that heroin was the most common drug injected, followed by cocaine. To curb the spread of HIV infection, the injection of both drugs must be curtailed.

Preliminary study results undertaken in shelters and hospitals show that AIDS is a major concern among shelter residents and that HIV infection has emerged as a major public health issue among homeless IVDUs. Further, the rates of any lifetime needle use and heroin addiction are greater among shelter residents and single-room-occupancy hotels than among residents of other types of accommodations.

Ethnographic and other studies reviewed, however, identify a group of addicts who avoid shelters or single-room-occupancy hotels and live primarily on the streets in abandoned buildings, subways, terminals, and other public places. Programs must be devised to reach these individuals if the AIDS epidemic is to be brought under control. Outreach units established through National Institute on Drug Abuse grants in six cities--New York, Philadelphia, Miami, Chicago, Houston, and San Francisco--are examining different approaches to outreach in various settings.

Preliminary research shows that addicts are aware that AIDS is transmitted through use of shared unsterilized needles. There are also indications that street addicts have attempted to reduce risk behavior by purchasing needles from dealers, attempting to clean needles, and sharing them less. Among homeless IVDUs, efforts at risk reduction appear to be difficult to sustain consistently. Outreach therefore must not only offer education but must also refer addicts to programs and services that will enable them to change deeply ingrained behavior that facilitates the transmission of the AIDS virus.

Homeless AIDS patients present serious medical management problems (e.g., lost to followup, failure to complete medical regimens, or long hospital stays). In addition, if they are not properly housed, they are subject to additional infection. Increases in the number of tuberculosis and syphilis cases reported to the New York City Department of Health during the past 2 years may be related to poverty, homelessness, and underlying HIV infection among IVDUs. To protect PWAs from further infection and the public from contagious diseases such as tuberculosis, proper housing for homeless IVDUs, especially those infected with the AIDS virus, is essential. The model housing programs developed for PWAs have limited capacities and cannot currently address the housing needs of this population.

Services should be established and evaluated near areas where homeless IVDUs congregate or in shelters or single-room-occupancy hotels. If possible, medical, social, and educational services should be combined into a single program rather than spread out in different locations. The value of onsite services is to help homeless patients follow through with medical or social service appointments and treatment procedures. For example, a high proportion of homeless men tested for HIV antibodies in New York City men's shelter reported for their test results. This service was offered in the shelter by the physicians who examined and counseled the patients.

The destruction of low-income housing in areas where drug abuse and AIDS are concentrated further exacerbates the dual conditions of poverty and homelessness, resulting in dispersal of the population most at risk for infection. The delivery of needed services and outreach are made more difficult because of the larger geographic area that must be served.

Another area of growing concern is the care of children born infected with the AIDS virus and the children of deceased AIDS patients. Based on current surveys, the number of newborns infected with the AIDS virus and the number of children needing placement will probably increase as more infected women who are IVDUs or sexual partners of men at risk become pregnant.

Historically, sharing unsterilized needles has resulted in serious public health problems. Diseases transmitted by addicts sharing needles include malaria, endocarditis, hepatitis, and AIDS. Although the legalization of needles and the establishment of needle exchanges to provide sterile needles to addicts are volatile issues, the future direction of the AIDS epidemic will be affected by the way these issues are resolved. A needle exchange program is currently in operation in Tacoma, Washington, and another will be created in New York City in November 1988. Both exchange programs are under the jurisdictions of the Departments of Health in the two cities. They will be evaluated over the next 2 years to determine whether they are effective.

There are an estimated 260,000 opiate addicts in New York State (New York State Division of Substance Abuse Services 1986). At present, about 38,000 addicts are in methadone programs (95 percent) and drug-free programs (5 percent). Since programs reach only 15 percent of the estimated addicts, expanding treatment for IV heroin addicts in New York State has now become a major public health effort. Outreach, however, is not sufficient. A sizeable number of addicts enter treatment only to drop out within a 2-year period, and most relapse. Therefore, long-term or even lifetime treatment for many homeless addicts would be necessary to curb the spread of HIV infection. Programs would have to encourage patients to remain in treatment for an indefinite period.

The programs and surveys presented in this chapter demonstrate that it is possible to reach out and assist a seemingly intractable population of homeless IVDUs. However, interventions are only a first step in changing lives and destructive behavior. Intervention without the backup of treatment, services, and housing can only lead to further despair, HIV infection, and other diseases among the homeless. At present, it is increasingly difficult to place individuals in programs. The most serious problems are the lack of adequate treatment facilities, housing for the homeless, and space to locate new programs. Community opposition to the establishment of both drug and AIDS treatment facilities and funding for services, including renovation and building of the necessary facilities, is common. Commitment, planning, and funds are needed to affect the spread of the AIDS virus within the homeless population.

Recommendations based on study of the programs and successful interventions discussed include the following:

(1) Sufficient program capacity should be developed and funded to reduce the waiting period for treatment and, if possible, eventually eliminate waiting lists. Clinic hours should be extended in existing programs, and medical centers that currently do not offer methadone treatment should develop such programs. The delivery, by vans, of methadone, bleach, condoms, and medication for treating cocaine users should be evaluated. However, to be effective in reducing transmission behavior, programs will have to address both IV heroin and cocaine abuse.

(2) Programs that specifically recruit homeless addicts for treatment using vans as intake and counseling offices should be implemented and expanded. Vans recruiting addicts for treatment in various neighborhoods make intake into treatment more accessible. The HEART Project, which aims at the homeless addict, brings knowledgeable workers to neighborhoods that may be isolated and that lack resources. This should be expanded.

(3) Frontline medical, social, and educational onsite services should be combined into a single program and developed at access points where addicts congregate and live (i.e., shelters, single-room-occupancy hotels, emergency rooms, criminal justice systems, and public health centers). Again, the delivery of medical and social services by vans to inaccessible populations should be investigated. Treatment and referral systems could be implemented at these access points, using the resources of several agencies to create new types of programs. KEEP, a program in the New York City jail system, is an excellent example of this type of intervention.

(4) Special residences and program components within existing residences should be developed for homeless substance abusers with AIDS that address treatment issues and monitor behavior in a humane, flexible manner. The facility should take into account the episodic nature of the illness

248

and accommodate patients who may require methadone maintenance, a drug-free approach, or special medication for pain or depression. The residence should offer a social support system similar to that in scatter-site housing, Bailey House, and Daytop Village. These models should be expanded. Funding should be earmarked for housing homeless PWAs under the provisions of the McKinney Act.

(5) Programs that combine chemotherapy in a residential setting should be developed for homeless IV drug abusers who may or may not be infected with the AIDS virus, but who are at risk for infection. The Short Stay Program, a residence for marginal methadone patients most of whom are homeless or on the verge of becoming homeless, is an example of this type of program.

(6) Outreach units that go into the streets, abandoned buildings, shooting galleries, shelters, jails, and single-room-occupancy and low-priced hotels to educate addicts about AIDS-related risk behavior and refer them to treatment should be expanded. The outreach program developed by ADAPT is a prime example of this program. Networks should be developed between outreach units and appropriate departments within medical centers to expedite referrals of homeless addicts to treatment programs, health facilities, and social service agencies.

(7) Medical centers should develop onsite programs for treating the homeless in shelters and furnished rooming houses. An example is the program administered by St. Vincent's Hospital at the Keener Shelter for Men on Ward's Island.

(8) Medical and social agencies dealing with this population must aggressively and cooperatively develop policies and programs aimed at containing the AIDS epidemic. Again, the KEEP program demonstrates what can be accomplished by three agencies with different but overlapping agendas (i.e., DSAS, Corrections, and Montefiore Hospital).

(9) The relationships between urban decay, the destruction of affordable low-income housing, and the spread of the AIDS epidemic should be investigated further.

(10) Evaluation of medical, social service, educational, outreach, and other possible programs should be conducted to determine program strengths and weaknesses.

REFERENCES

Brickner, P.W. Department of Community Medicine, St. Vincent's Hospital, New York City. Personal communication, 1988.

Brickner, P.W.; Scanlan, B.C.; Conanan, B.; et al. Homeless Persons and Health Care. *Ann Int Med* 104(3):405-409, 1986.

Brown, L. ARTC, New York City. Personal communication, 1987.

Bureau of Chemotherapy Services. New York State Division of Substance Abuse Services. *Waiting List Summary Sheet*, February 1988.

City Health Information. *Tuberculosis and Acquired Immunodeficiency Syndrome in New York City: Special AIDS Issue #1.* New York City Department of Health, March 1988.

Deren, S. Principal Investigator, Harlem AIDS Outreach and Demonstration Project, NDRI, Inc., New York, NY. Personal communication, 1988.

Des Jarlais, D.C. Coordinator of AIDS Research, New York State Division of Substance Abuse Services. Personal communication, 1988.

Des Jarlais, D.; Friedman, S.R.; and Hopkins, W. Risk reduction for the acquired immunodeficiency syndrome among intravenous drug users. *Ann Int Med* 103(5):755-759, 1985.

Des Jarlais, D., and Hopkins, W. "Free" needles for intravenous drug users at risk for AIDS: Current developments in New York City. *N Engl J Med* 313(23):1476, 1985.

Drucker, E. Montefiore Hospital. Personal communication 1988.

Fenlon, V. Management Information System, New York State Division of Substance Abuse Services. Personal communication, 1988.

Fisher, E. *Housing for Homeless People With AIDS in New York City.* AIDS Resource Center, Inc., 24 West 30th Street, New York, NY 10001, January 1988.

Fisher, E. AIDS Resource Center. Personal communication, 1988.

Frank, B.; Hopkins, W.; and Maranda, M. *Homeless Drug Abusers in New York City: A Hidden Population.* New York State Division of Substance Abuse Services, Treatment Issue Report No. 54, 1985.

Friedman, S. Principal Investigator, AIDS Community Outreach Demonstration Project, Narcotic Drug and Research, Inc., New York City. Personal communication, 1988.

Haig, M. Beth Israel Medical Center AIDS Coordinator. Personal communication, 1988.

Haugh, G., Director of Bailey House. Personal communication, 1988.

Hopkins, W. Director of Street Unit, New York State Division of Substance Abuse Services. Personal communication, 1988.

Hopkins, W. Needle sharing and street behavior in response to AIDS in New York City. In: Battjes, R., and Pickens, R., eds. *Needle Sharing Among Intravenous Drug Users: National and International Perspectives*. National Institute on Drug Abuse Research, Monograph 80. DHHS Pub. No. (ADM)88-1567. Washington, DC: Supt. of Docs., U.S. Govt. Print. Off., 1988. pp. 18-23.

Joseph, H.; Appel, P.; Marx, R.; Perez, J.; Tardelo, F.; and Watts, L. *Evaluation of Pre-KEEP in Three Facilities of the New York City Department of Corrections on Rikers Island*. New York: New York State Division of Substance Abuse Services, Bureau of Research and Evaluation, 1988.

Joseph, S. Commissioner, New York City Department Health. News release, April 16, 1988.

Kolata, G. Many with AIDS said to live in shelters in New York City. *New York Times*, April 4, 1988, p. B1.

Magura, S. Narcotic Drug and Research, Inc., New York City. Personal communication, 1987.

Management Information System. *Summary Management Report of Clients in Treatment Programs*. New York: New York State Division of Substance Abuse Services, 1988.

Mauge, C. Director, AIDS Outreach Project. Personal communication, 1988.

Mayberry, E. Administrative Director, Division of Foster Care, Human Resources Administration. Personal communication, 1988.

McAdam, J. Department of Community Medicine, St. Vincent's Hospital. Personal communication, 1988.

New York City Department of Health. *AIDS Surveillance Update*. AIDS Surveillance Unit. February 1988a.

New York City Department of Health. *Annual Tuberculosis Report*. New York: the Department, 1988b.

New York State Department of Health. *AIDS in New York State*. New York: the Department, 1988.

New York State Division of Substance Abuse Services. *State Comprehensive Five-Year Plan, Third Annual Update*. New York: the Division, 1986.

New York State Division of Substance Abuse Services. *Summary Management Report of Clients in Treatment Programs*. New York: the Division, February 1988.

New York State Division of Substance Abuse Services Bureau of Chemotherapy Services. *Waiting List Report for Methadone Programs.* New York: the Division, 1988.

Partnership for the Homeless. *Assisting the Homeless in New York City: A Review of the Last Year and Challenges for 1988.* New York Partnership for the Homeless, 1988a.

Partnership for the Homeless. News release, December 1, 1988b.

Perowsky, P. Personal communication, 1988.

Pittman, J. Epidemiology of Mental Disorders Research Department, Community Support Systems Evaluation Program, New York State Psychiatric Institute. Personal communication, 1988.

Serrano, Y. ADAPT. Personal communication, 1988.

Sorrell, S. Daytop Village and Roosevelt Hospital, New York City. Personal communication, 1988.

Springer, E. ADAPT. Personal communication, 1988.

Stoneburner, R.; Des Jarlais, D.; and Friedman, S. Increasing mortality among IV drug users. Presented at the 115th Annual Meeting of the American Public Health Association, October 24, 1987.

Struening, E.L. New York State Psychiatric Institute. Personal communication, 1988.

Struening, E.L., and Pittman, J. *Characteristics of Residents of the New York City Shelter System: Executive Summary.* New York: New York State Psychiatric Institute, 1988.

Torres, R.A. Department of Community Medicine, St. Vincent's Hospital. Personal communication, 1988.

Torres, R.A.; Lefkowitz, P.; Kales, C.; and Brickner, P.W. Homelessness among hospitalized patients with the acquired immunodeficiency syndrome in New York City. *JAMA* 258:779-780, 1987.

Triscari, A. Division of AIDS Services, Human Resources Administration. Personal communication, 1988.

Wallace, R. Research Scientist, New York State Psychiatric Institute. Personal communication, 1988.

Wallace, R. A synergism of plagues: Planned shrinkages, contagious housing destruction and AIDS in the Bronx. *Environ Res* 47, in press.

Wender, M. Assistant Coordinator, AIDS Resource Unit, New York State Division of Substance Abuse Services. Personal communication, 1988.

Woods, J. Director, Keener Shelter for Men. Personal communication, 1988.

AUTHORS

Herman Joseph
Research Scientist
Bureau of Research
    and Evaluation

Hilda Roman-Nay, J.D.
Director
Bureau of Government
    and Community Relations

The Homeless Project
State of New York Division of Substance Abuse Services
55 West 125th Street, 10th Floor
New York, NY 10027

HIV-Related Disorders, Needle Users, and the Social Services

Lawrence C. Shulman, Joanne E. Mantell,
Charles Eaton, and Stephan Sorrell

INTRODUCTION

With the increasing rates of acquired immunodeficiency syndrome (AIDS) in the United States among intravenous drug users (IVDUs), their sex partners, and their children, intensive prevention and control efforts are needed to curb the spread of the epidemic. IVDUs comprise the second largest risk group for AIDS in the United States and, in New York City, account for more than half of all AIDS-related mortality. They are the major link to spreading the human immunodeficiency virus (HIV) beyond groups with defined high-risk behaviors. The reported number of women who contracted AIDS through heterosexual transmission more than doubled since 1982 (from 12 percent to 30 percent) (Guinan and Hardy 1987; Centers for Disease Control 1988). Since 1981, more than 21,000 IVDUs (27 percent of the cumulative number of AIDS cases nationwide) have been reported with a diagnosis of AIDS. Recent data in New York City and San Francisco indicate that rates of HIV infection are increasing among IVDUs who inject cocaine exclusively (Lambert 1988a). In New York City, the proportion of IVDUs with AIDS is substantially higher, representing 38.3 percent of all New York City cumulative adult cases (New York City Department of Health 1989). A recent review of narcotic-related deaths on New York City death certificates, which were then matched to the New York City Department of Health AIDS Surveillance Registry data, indicates that AIDS has been grossly underreported (Stoneburner et al. 1988). Narcotics-related deaths increased on the average of 32 percent a year between 1981 (n=492) and 1986 (n=1996). Although many of these deaths among IVDUs did not meet the AIDS surveillance case definition, many were caused by conditions suggestive of HIV infection, such as unspecified pneumonia, endocarditis, and tuberculosis (TB).

HIV infection rates vary widely across the Nation, with rates as high as 50 to 60 percent in New York, New Jersey, and Puerto Rico to less than 5 percent in areas outside the east coast (Centers for Disease Control 1987). The National Institute on Drug Abuse estimates that of the 1.1 million IVDUs in the United States, 335,000 are infected with HIV. New York City has 50 percent of the needle-using, opiate-dependent (heroin, street methadone, pharmaceutical) population in the United States, and IVDUs now surpass homosexual/bisexual men as the major group with AIDS.

The mounting numbers of AIDS cases due to intravenous (IV), intramuscular, and subcutaneous drug use are straining the health and social service delivery systems, especially the drug treatment sector. Resources for both drug and AIDS-related treatment are drastically inadequate. In this chapter, we use the term "needle drug user" (NDU) to indicate more appropriately the range of risk behaviors implicated in HIV transmission.

CONCEPTUAL FRAMEWORK OF THE SOCIAL SERVICE SYSTEM

Definition and Models of Social Services

Social services may be viewed as efforts to support, supplement, and substitute for functions traditionally performed by the family or as efforts to provide supports to compensate for the individual and family dislocations caused by roller-coaster economic forces (Shulman 1985). Social services are provided within the framework of human service organizations and are charged with enhancing physical, economic, and psychosocial well-being. Contemporary social welfare activity encompasses a wide range of organized services, entitlements (insurances), and institutions that are "designed to aid individuals and groups to attain satisfying standards of life and health" (Brager and Hollaway 1978). While specialization in social services delivery can lead to efficiency, it also fosters fragmentation of the client or family unit, lack of coordination, gaps and duplication in service delivery, and client stigmatization.

Traditionally, social services have been organized along either a residual or institutional conceptual model (Wilensky and Lebeaux 1965). Throughout history, social policy, planning, and service design have been directly affected (and expanded or contracted) by the prevailing ethos and the sociopolitical climate. The resulting system is a patchwork of laws, regulations, and public voluntary and self-help agencies and services. The residual model emphasizes self-reliance, economic individualism, and moralistic judgment regarding responsibility for one's actions and the potential consequences of "antisocial" or "deviant" behaviors. The institutional model sees social welfare services as the required base or "safety net" to support vulnerable or at-risk persons, families, or groups in a highly fluid, cyclical modern industrial society (Brager and Hollaway 1978).

Agencies, programs, and services developed with the residual model as a conceptual or philosophical base tend to erect eligibility barriers and provide the services in ways perceived to be hostile by the NDU population. These agencies are not designed to reach out or accommodate the psychological and social fluctuations that characterize the lifestyles of the NDU and family. The institutional model, on the other hand, is generally less judgmental of the individual, but, by the nature of large-scale entitlement or safety net programs, agencies organized along this conceptual framework tend to blend the individual-in-crisis into a standardized category.

All agencies serving the NDU population have struggled for decades with their level of social responsibility for service delivery to people with chemical dependency disorders, as well as with shifting concepts of treatment. The patchwork of public and private programs and funding has not fostered a coherent, coordinated planning or treatment approach.

The funding, organization, and delivery of social services to addicts with AIDS must be examined within the context of episodic hospitalizations, shortened survival, and the interactive effect of multiple chronic health problems. General problems of surviving as an addict are heightened immeasurably by the presence of HIV infection.

Underlying lifestyle factors, such as poverty, unstable family structures, and overall high-risk environment, further compound an NDU's access to and use of social services. New York City has been especially hard hit by the epidemic of HIV infection among drug users (47 percent of all cases diagnosed since January 1, 1988), many of whom lack health insurance and other supportive resources (New York City Department of Health 1989).

Service Delivery Interface

NDUs may interface with the service provider industry in one or more of the following categories:

- Public assistance (home relief)

- Medicaid program

- Social Security/Social Security (wage-related) disability

- Unemployment program

- Child welfare service

- Supplemental Security Income program

- Law enforcement system (police, court officers, judges, corrections officers, parole officers, Drug Enforcement Agency personnel, Legal Aid staff, and Legal Services programs)

- Hospital and health department clinics

- Psychiatric clinics and outreach programs, psychiatric inpatient units

- Shelters

- Meal programs

- Drug treatment programs such as drug-free residential and ambulatory therapeutic communities, and community-based methadone maintenance treatment programs

- Social agencies (especially programs for runaway youth)

A NEW YORK CITY VOLUNTARY HOSPITAL AND THE SERVICE DELIVERY INTERFACE

St. Luke's-Roosevelt Hospital Center has had an active Substance Abuse Program (SAP) funded through patient reimbursement mechanisms for the past 17 years and has provided methadone treatment to more than 4,000 patients cumulatively. The clinic provides treatment 6 days a week. The hospital also has both

257

inpatient alcohol and drug detoxification units. About 12 new patients are admitted to the SAP each month. Many of the patients on methadone maintenance are multiple substance abusers; 65 percent are male; 35 percent of the patients are Hispanic; 32 percent are white; and another 31 percent are black. Patients range in age from 19 to 74 years. Medicaid recipients make up 46 percent of the population, and 35 percent of the SAP clientele are employed either parttime or fulltime. Between 1984 and 1986, approximately 36 percent of the patients who requested antibody testing were HIV seropositive (Grieco 1988), and, as of April 1987, 36.7 percent were seropositive (Sorrell, personal communication, 1988).

Substance abusers (and their children) are seen in all of our ambulatory and inpatient services, including the emergency department, obstetrical/gynecological clinics, and pediatric clinics. Many enter our health care system in crisis, requiring the mobilization of protective social services, entitlement assistance and advocacy, legal referrals, and housing or income maintenance. The Hospital Center has a well-trained, professional Department of Social Work whose social workers and drug counselors provide aggressive counseling and referral services to this population. In addition, the Department of Social Work established a Public Entitlements Program to provide advocacy assistance to patients and staff in overcoming barriers to accessing services required by all patients of the hospital. Even with the availability of these expert Entitlement Specialists, many social and health services cannot be obtained for the substance abuse population because of constraints and limitations within the broader service delivery system. Many of the observations and recommendations in this paper are drawn from our experience at St. Luke's-Roosevelt as well as from other service providers in the field of substance abuse.

More recently, extensive work with IVDUs and their families has occurred in our AIDS Center Program. The multiple needs and increasing proportion of cases among this population-at-risk has caused the hospital, the Department of Social Work, and the SAP to reexamine the ways in which health and social services are delivered to the NDU population within the hospital programs. For example, we considered the establishment of a special inpatient AIDS unit for NDUs to evaluate the effectiveness of clinical care and social work services. Two trained drug counselors were hired to provide liaison, education, and prevention services to the hospitalized NDU population. Social work staff assigned to AIDS services has tripled since September 1987 (8 master's level social workers for an average inpatient census of 85 in 1988).

The hospital has developed an education and prevention outreach program for street prostitutes and runaway youth in its geographic area who are at high risk for HIV infection because of drug use and multiple sex partners. Staff will be assigned to street work in cooperation with three community-based organizations to link drug abusers to the social services system, to advocate for needed entitlements, to encourage prostitutes to seek HIV counseling and testing, and to encourage and refer clients to enter drug and health treatment programs. Our goal is to develop a low-barrier, nontraditional primary health care service for women, their children, male prostitutes, and street youth involved in the dual cycle of sex and drugs.

BARRIERS TO SERVICE DELIVERY

Barriers to access and utilization of services by NDUs are evident in the areas of service delivery design, client resistance, public and staff attitudes and beliefs, and public policy.

An observer will quickly discern that social agency program procedures and policies are not geared to the needs of NDUs. All too often, agencies develop and enact regulations and procedures that result in systems maintenance and that meet staff and administrative imperatives rather than meeting client needs (Goffman 1967). The resistant behaviors of drug users and the deficits in the service delivery system compound the problems of the AIDS epidemic and its link to needle-associated HIV transmission.

Service providers who perceive that NDUs are socially marginal and unable to change their behaviors--that is, once an addict, always an addict--may have antagonistic dealings with clients and their families. These attitudes reinforce the resistant behaviors of both clients and the social services system by creating an unwelcome climate that does not provide "user friendly" services.

Public policy has treated drug abuse historically as a criminal rather than a health or social problem. Drug control and drug interdiction have received greater public and governmental support than drug treatment approaches or social problem solutions. With the intertwining of AIDS, drug abuse, and crime, however, pressure to

259

expand drug treatment programs is accelerating (Kerr 1988; Lambert 1988b).

The NDU is the uncontrolled link to widespread drug-related HIV transmission, as well as sexual and perinatal HIV transmission, and thus represents the explosive potential for spread of the disease. Since AIDS is disproportionally represented by two stigmatized risk groups (gay men and IVDUs), the "victims" are blamed and the need for social services basically ignored. Only when sensational claims of "dire threat to the heterosexual population" or the irrational fear of casual contagion receive high media visibility does the need for public spending and resource allocation become recognized (Check 1987). St. Luke's-Roosevelt Hospital staff and other drug treatment program staff report that, historically, NDUs have been cut off in a real sense from formal health and social service organizations. Their longstanding, inherent characterological problems in living and manipulation of "the system" mirrors their difficulty in dealing appropriately with all aspects of their lives. Needle users with HIV-related disease enter the mainstream health care and social service systems in a more advanced stage of disease than do gay men or people with transfusion-associated disease (Maayan et al. 1985; Belmont et al. 1985). Moreover, as reflected by New York City AIDS-related mortality data, IVDUs (especially black females), have the poorest survival from diagnosis to death compared to people with other risk-associated behaviors (Rothenberg et al. 1987).

Unlike the "junkiebonden," the junkie unions in The Netherlands, which are collective self-help organizations set up by drug users, needle users in the United States generally lack the natural or shared community evident in organized self-identified gay populations where there is active political and social advocacy for their constituents. Needle users are frequently economically and socially disadvantaged. Based on our experience at St. Luke's-Roosevelt Hospital Center, we suggest that for nondrug-using female partners of NDUs, the additional barrier of economic dependence on the NDU male partner may limit access to formal services, because of the NDUs' suspicious-ness and distrust of authority. Concrete problems of day-to-day survival in families where one or both partners use drugs are intensified and complicated by AIDS.

Psychological factors can be a barrier to service delivery. Empirical and anecdotal data from drug treatment centers revealed temporary drug bingeing following notification to the addict of positive HIV antibody status (Marlink et al. 1987). Real and/or perceived social

260

stigmatization about being a "two-time loser" (a drug addict and an infected HIV carrier) may also act as a barrier to service use.

Few social service programs have been established to serve NDUs on a priority basis. Funding has supported methadone and drug-free treatment centers to the exclusion of other social services that are crucial to the rehabilitation of the drug addict. Even the availability of drug treatment "slots" has been far below the acknowledged need level. About 100,000 treatment slots are available nationwide, or spaces for about 1 out of 12 addicts (*New York Times* 1988a). In New York City, for example, residential drug treatment programs offer fewer than 6,000 spaces, methadone maintenance treatment programs (MMTPs) have 29,000 addicts enrolled, and another 10,000 addicts are in community-based drug-free programs. New York has an estimated 200,000 drug addicts. Many desire treatment and are turned away and placed on waiting lists.

Until recently, there was major opposition to permitting distribution of free needles and syringes to addicts in New York City. Societal resistance to this revolutionary proposal stems, in part, from the unwillingness to challenge public drug and law enforcement officials' beliefs that provision of clean needles condones and legitimizes drug use and abets an illegal activity. A free needle distribution campaign is contrary to the ideology of therapeutic drug-free communities, which view sobriety as the primary value. Data from The Netherlands, France, England, Scotland, and Tacoma, WA, show that, with governmental distribution of free needles and syringes, significant numbers of NDUs are exchanging their syringes and needle-sharing practices have decreased (Balian et al. 1988; Mulleady et al. 1988; Gross 1989).

The unavailability of appropriate and adequate housing is a problem for many people with HIV-related disorders, but for addicts who are diagnosed late, the problems are exacerbated. As many NDUs do not have intact social support systems, they do not have family and friends to assume caregiving responsibilities in the home. Caring for addicts with symptomatic HIV infection is almost impossible in a context of homelessness. An ineffective support system is further compromised by their poor health status. If an NDU is unable to maintain self-care, home care options are limited, and residential-based models of health and social service delivery become essential. Public shelters in New York City do not knowingly accept persons with AIDS. When families of the NDUs with HIV-related disorders are also homeless, the housing crisis is worsened.

Substance abuse treatment is generally unresponsive to the needs of women. Women do not have adequate network support to motivate them to enter treatment. Treatment models tend to be male-oriented, and case-finding systems are not gender-sensitive (Mondanaro 1989). Few agencies have programs for pregnant addicts or deal with issues of child care, foster care, parenting education, job retraining, and limited ability to pay for treatment (Cohen et al., in press). In New York City, 1 in 61 babies are born HIV seroposi-tive, and in the Bronx, 1 in 43, statistics that coincide with endemic areas of high drug use in the city (Novick et al. 1988). Over 100 "boarder babies" were reportedly abandoned in New York City hospi-tals in 1987, because they were infected or their families were too sick to care for them. While availability of foster care placement for such infants has increased in New York City, there are few other alternatives when a mother or family members are unable to provide at-home care.

Two recent studies attribute social factors as the cause of children's unnecessary medical hospitalizations. At Yale-New Haven Hospital in Connecticut, 54 percent (n=18) of 34 children with symptoms of HIV infection remained in the hospital beyond medical need (Kemper and Forsyth 1988). Difficulty in placement was associated with a dis-organized home environment due to parental IV drug use, hospitaliza-tion or jail placement, or death. Similarly, a Harlem Hospital Study in New York City found that 86 percent of the parents of the 37 children with AIDS-related complex (ARC) or AIDS were NDUs. Many of the unnecessary hospitalizations were attributed to unstable family life; children with less serious health problems had the same amount of hospital medical costs as those who were seriously ill or had died (Heagarty et al. 1988).

FRAMEWORK FOR SOCIAL SERVICE SYSTEMS PLANNING AND POLICY DEVELOPMENT

Strategic planning, with a needs-assessment component, provides a useful framework for the design and delivery of comprehensive social services for people with HIV-spectrum disorders. First, there must be recognition of the diversity of NDUs. The needs of the homeless NDU, the adolescent addict, street prostitutes who support their habit as sex industry workers, heroin addicts, skin-popping addicts, those on methadone maintenance, and those in drug-free treatment pro-grams must be distinguished. These differences suggest that multiple points of access, different social service models, and various channels of service delivery will be required to reach subsets of the population.

Second, the fit between service providers' characteristics and those of the NDU group needs to be examined. What cultural, language, ethnic, and socioeconomic barriers might interfere with service provision and utilization?

Third, family influence on the use of social and health services must be addressed. How does the codependency of some family members impede service use? Social service delivery systems need to develop ways to build upon the strengths of the family to support and reinforce the addict's psychosocial and medical "treatment" plan.

Finally, the pathways and procedures surrounding the matrix of public and private sector services and entitlements and the messages that they convey to potential service recipients require critical examination.

CONSIDERATIONS FOR DESIGNING AND DELIVERING SOCIAL SERVICES

The heterogeneity and complexity of social, medical, psychological, and economic needs of the NDU population, coupled with the rapid spread of HIV infection among NDUs and their sex partners, suggest that we can no longer be rigidly wedded to existing service delivery structures. Provision of social services between 9 a.m. and 5 p.m. may be convenient to staff, but not necessarily responsive to clients' lifestyles and variable health conditions.

Integration of Health Services and Social Services for the NDU Population

Models for service delivery to the NDU population require effective integration of those complex components of care: health, drug treatment services, social services, including housing, income supports, maternal and child health and nutrition services, disability supports, job programs, and legal and advocacy services. Community planning and coordinating efforts are a first step in the development of such models. Organizing and nurturing community coalitions, such as the New York AIDS Coalition and the Worcester AIDS Consortium (Massachusetts), is needed to develop a consensus and support base for addressing the broad range of problems facing NDUs.

The fragmented organization and lack of continuity of health and social services existed prior to the epidemic of HIV infection. With the burgeoning numbers of infected drug users, the epidemic has exacerbated these gaps by placing excessive strains on service systems and creating a shortage of personnel resources. The coalition of agencies in Worcester monitors HIV surveillance, facilitates priority entry of clients into drug treatment, and provides risk-reduction services (distributing bleach and condoms) (Lewis et al. 1988).

Low-Barrier Models

Developing low-barrier access to social service systems to increase service use must be considered. Social services should be designed and provided in a way that increases the trust of HIV-infected addicts and their families. In addition, entitlement system requirements that erect barriers to service accessibility must be reexamined. Similarly, Federal regulations that require methadone clinics to provide addicts with counseling (as part of treatment) place another barrier in the pathway of those desiring treatment and drive addicts away from mainstream service facilities.

Four low-barrier social services models suggested for evaluation are:

(1)　Mobile (van) services with a multidisciplinary team of medical, case management, and prevention staff would provide more direct access to NDUs. Mobile services would be concentrated in communities with high HIV-related mortality rates and would be satellites of acute health care facilities.

(2)　Storefront multipurpose service centers, like those developed by the Office of Economic Opportunity in the 1960s, could be set up to bring services closer to addicts. Storefront facilities, coupled with effective case management, may help break down barriers between addicts and the system.

(3)　Low-barrier drop-in service centers where NDUs could receive services with minimal or no requirements could try to reach the difficult-to-access addict who shuns the formal treatment and service systems.

(4)　Outreach workers/teams that go "where the action is"--on the street, in neighborhood hangouts, and shooting galleries. This approach is similar to that used by the New York City Youth

Board in the late 1950s and early 1960s to work with youth gangs and has been used by the Association for Drug Abuse Prevention and Treatment, Inc., in New York City and by ethnographic field workers in San Francisco, CA; Chicago, IL; Baltimore, MD; New York City; Washington, DC; El Paso, TX; and others.

The underlying thrust of each of these four models is to bring social services to the community--to remove barriers to service accessibility and availability. These recommended service models are based on experiential understanding that NDUs and their families (1) tend to be suspicious of and avoid "official" public social agencies (unless absolutely necessary for survival), and (2) are resistant to using highly bureaucratic service agencies that present eligibility and utilization barriers.

Case Management Strategies

Effective and realistic case management strategies for NDUs with HIV-related disorders must be developed. Continuity of care is essential for AIDS-diagnosed addicts and their families, who move rapidly between hospitalization, drug treatment, social service agencies, their homes, and, in some cases, the streets. While providing a single case manager for these clients may be unrealistic, the multiple case management systems these clients encounter must be coordinated, with all (including the NDU) agreeing upon who should be the primary case manager. Linkage and coordination with formal and informal community-based institutions are necessary. Intensive efforts must also be directed toward strengthening links with public entitlement systems and perhaps broadening their scope of responsibilities as well. For example, in New York City, the Health Resources Administration formed an AIDS Case Management Unit to deal with public assistance and Medicaid needs of persons with AIDS and funds a residential facility for homeless persons with AIDS (Campbell, personal communication, 1987). Links with community-based institutions, such as schools, churches, welfare, vocational rehabilitation, day care, foster care, prisons, and juvenile justice systems, must be forged.

Provision of Concrete and Clinical Services

Direct provision of concrete social services might attract NDUs to an AIDS education and counseling program. Services might include HIV antibody counseling and testing, screening for sexually transmitted diseases (STDs) and TB, and service advocacy, especially legal, hous-ing, and public assistance. The provision of these services might increase NDUs' tolerance and tentative trust of the professional health care providers. For example, the AWARE program for sex industry workers in San Francisco has found the provision of a health and physical evaluation, and HIV counseling and antibody testing, are effective means of engaging and maintaining women in the program (Cohen, personal communication, 1987).

Provision of mental health services for NDUs with HIV-spectrum disorders and their collaterals is essential. Currently, there are few psychosocial support services available for the asymptomatic sero-positive; day treatment services for those suffering from impaired mental functioning as a result of AIDS dementia are virtually nonexistent. Treatment services for children whose parents or siblings have AIDS are only just being developed in some communities.

Greater creativity and innovation in the use of volunteers and indigenous staff to support the NDU with AIDS are essential. A corps of indigenous public health and social service workers who are recovering addicts must be recruited and trained to work in the high-risk, high-drug-activity areas. These "natural" helpers serve as gatekeepers of the community and can help bridge the gap between the NDUs and the formal health and social service institutions.

Intensive community outreach with "shooting gallery" and "crack-house" owners or managers should be attempted and evaluated to examine the potential for reaching untreated addicts. Owners may be trained to urge addicts to take advantage of the new social services being provided. In addition, if needle exchange programs were to move beyond the pilot demonstration phase, they could serve as the gatekeepers for needles and "works" exchanges.

Increased Drug Treatment Resources

The availability, accessibility, and adequacy of drug treatment are core ingredients of a comprehensive social service system for NDUs. While funding for 5,000 more methadone treatment slots has been approved in New York City, the numbers will still be inadequate to handle the 50,000 spaces needed to accommodate the influx of addicts desiring treatment (Schmalz 1988). Some expansion could be handled by extending the hours of treatment programs and converting city-owned buildings into drug treatment facilities to serve an additional 3,000 addicts (*New York Times* 1988b).

Residential programs that provide treatment for substance abuse disorders and AIDS and case management for NDUs with AIDS are essential. Not all NDUs with HIV-related disease can function independently and be managed on an outpatient service basis for sociomedical care. A variety of institutional arrangements will be required. Several drug treatment programs are moving beyond their traditional roles and attempting to establish innovative residential services for addicts with ARC or AIDS. For example, San Francisco's Baker Places has opened a daytime six-bed cooperative care unit for people with triple diagnoses—ARC/AIDS, substance abuse, and a DSM Axis 1 or 2 psychiatric disorder—and plans to open a 21-bed residential treatment unit for those capable of independent living in the near future (Vernick, personal communication, 1987). Samaritan Village and Project Return, large, drug-free therapeutic communities (TCs) in New York City, have embarked upon a joint project to set up an extended substance abuse treatment program within a TC environment for HIV-symptomatic recovering addicts (Barton, personal communication, 1988). These facilities might function like a flexible health-related facility or an intermediate care facility, but provisions would have to be made for maintaining a fixed number of skilled nursing-level beds.

Combining Models in a Multiservice "Bridging" Project

The recently begun Pilot Needle Exchange Study of the New York City Department of Health provides an example of integration of health services and social services for the NDU population. NDUs who want drug abuse treatment, but who cannot be immediately admitted, can obtain services from the Department of Health through the efforts of outreach workers or the treatment programs themselves. The staff of the Needle Exchange Study develop individualized case management strategies as a "bridge to treatment." These strategies induce health services, STD tests and HIV antibody testing, counseling on risk reduction for both sexual and needle-sharing routes of transmission, and advocacy to obtain the earliest possible entry into treatment.

Housing Alternatives

The lack of viable community-based alternatives to acute care has resulted in excessive overstay of patients in acute care facilities, as well as an inadequate number of appropriate housing facilities across the spectrum of need. In New York City, these patients are likely to be NDUs. While there is a serious lack of nursing homes and hospice care, there are also inadequate services for persons with AIDS (PWAs) who need a lower level of housing/supportive care. Many residential care facilities do not want to accept the PWA with a history of NDU because of management problems, e.g., how to handle patients who have not kicked the habit and "shoot up" on the premises. Discrimination and fear, the NIMBY (not in my backyard) syndrome in the community, also play a major part in restricting the development of housing resources. The lack of health insurance, difficulty in securing public entitlements, and lack of documentation to prove public assistance/Medicaid eligibility are major barriers to the NDU obtaining supportive housing. To date, there have been few successful housing initiatives for persons with HIV-related illness.

Homelessness has increasingly become a problem among persons with HIV-related disorders. NDUs with HIV infection may lose their housing because of difficulty in accessing the social services system, money mismanagement, disorganized lifestyles, health complications or activities of daily living problems, and discrimination (Norman 1988). In many urban areas, especially where there is a large low-income population, adequate, affordable housing is most difficult to obtain and is a major cause of homelessness. For the NDUs, especially those infected with HIV, the problem of housing accessibility is compounded.

While there are many unresolved questions pertaining to the most effective and appropriate housing alternatives for NDUs, we recommend that experimental, innovative solutions be tested for housing addicts and their families. This might include emergency housing vouchers (Froner 1988), the provision of onsite methadone with counseling and job-related services as well as a minimal service program that provides methadone to those waiting for acceptance into treatment programs (such as the outpatient program of New York's Beth Israel Medical Center recently approved by the Food and Drug Administration). Since private real estate interests have been slow to participate in developing housing resources for NDUs and the homeless, it will become the responsibility of public social services and the not-for-profit social agency sector to mobilize the resources and serve as catalysts in establishing these programs. One such program that could serve as a model for public/voluntary partnership is the San Francisco Department of Health's AIDS/ARC residential program for the homeless population (many of whom have substance abuse and/or mental health problems), which provides housing, social services, nursing care, and family counseling (Carpi 1988; San Francisco Department of Health 1988).

The specialized needs of women with AIDS and the increasing population of HIV-infected babies of parents who are NDUs must be addressed. Respite care for the mother or regular caregiver is one arrangement that might increase a family's ability to remain intact. Housing and cooperative care for mothers who may be sick with HIV, but want to keep their babies, is critical. For families unable to care for their children, hospice programs (home based, hospital based or freestanding) should be considered. Health services, income supports or supplementation, and psychosocial support services may also be required.

Reaching Youth At Risk

While less than 1 percent (n=325) of all reported AIDS cases have occurred among adolescents as of December 12, 1988 (Centers for Disease Control 1988), 21 percent (n=16,662) are among persons between the ages of 20 and 29 years. Many of the latter were probably infected during their teens as it may take up to 8 years between the time of infection and the onset of HIV illness. Adolescents who lead dysfunctional or disorganized lives are at higher risk for HIV infection than is currently evident in epidemiological data. They reflect a spectrum of youth including: (1) the growing number of runaways who show up in major cities and get involved in drugs, crime, and prostitution; (2) homeless youth who are part of homeless families; (3) hard-core unemployed youth; (4) adolescents who are heavily into polydrug abuse or hustling activities; and sexually abused teens (Daley 1988; Axthelm 1988). Of the approximately 1 million teenagers who run away each year, 187,500 are estimated to be involved in drug use, drug trafficking, prostitution, or solicitation (U.S. Department of Health and Human Services 1986). In addition, many adolescents who are still functional at home and in school are experimenting with drugs and sex. These adolescents are difficult to engage, because they are alienated from the mainstream service delivery system. Therefore, strategies must be developed to reach them within the context of their "natural" communities—in schools, at "hang-outs," on the streets, bus terminals, rock concerts, and record/video stores. Offers of food, shelter, clothing, and pocket money may be necessary to approach adolescents and "break the ice."

While adolescence is a turbulent, distrustful developmental stage under the best of circumstances, when compounded by drug abuse, the prospects for effective service engagement are diminished. Therefore, innovative "offbeat" ways must be devised to make services available and inviting to kids who "hang tough." Outreach services sponsored by community organizations should be linked with discrete, creatively designed school, hospital, clinic-based, or mobile health services to make care more accessible.

The social and health services systems need to recognize and deal with the conflict between adolescent resistance to parent-guided utilization of services and the lack of emancipated minor status of many youth. Issues of insurance and reimbursement for services under public or private systems must be resolved to improve delivery of services to this population (Hein 1988).

RESEARCH RECOMMENDATIONS

All the social service initiatives discussed in the previous section must be supported by planned, systematic process, outcome, and impact evaluation to determine program effectiveness and outcomes. All-too-many programs have been designed and implemented based on professional intuition or common wisdom and have lacked an effective evaluation component. Program and education/prevention strategies that show promise in reducing HIV infection rates and/or slowing the spread of AIDS, increasing addicts' entry into drug treatment, and their use of health and social services, must be explored.

- Needs assessment

  Needs assessment is a formative type of evaluation used to help shape population-sensitive and service-effective social service and health programs.

  The design of innovative and nontraditional programs must be supported by a documentation of the needs of the various subsets of the NDU populations. For example, the health and social service needs of drug-using street prostitutes may not be the same as those of a hard-core crackhouse population. A needs assessment may inform us that these employed women require ongoing monitoring of health status and STDs, child care

270

assistance, and psychosocially supportive services. Such assessment might lead us to the development of a low-barrier primary care health and social services center (like a storefront).

In contrast, the single male homeless addict might be shown to require residential drug treatment as a means to extricate himself from the destructive and seductive street environment.

- Program evaluation

  Evaluation of traditional and low-barrier services to the NDU population is essential. Dedicated resources for outreach services to NDUs are both labor and resource intensive. For example, the use of a mobile van to provide multipurpose HIV prevention services and case management must be evaluated to determine whether the delivery of services in this fashion is more effective than providing them in a traditional institutional setting. Evaluation would assess the numbers of people served, staff/client ratio, number of counseling sessions required to engage a client, number of referrals made to social service and drug treatment agencies, number of entitlement Fair Hearings held, etc. Program impact evaluation would entail assessment of changes in NDU clients' HIV-related knowledge, attitudes, and behaviors. The success of program outcome might be measured by a reduction of HIV sero-prevalence and STD rates among NDUs in the broader community.

  Another example of needed evaluation research relates to the current controversy over the relative effectiveness of providing methadone alone on demand to NDUs awaiting entry into treatment programs versus methadone provided as part of a comprehensive chemical dependency program that involves psychotherapy, residential milieu treatment, vocational counseling, and job-finding services.

  Assessment of the effectiveness of community outreach workers as "natural helpers" for HIV risk-reduction education and linkage to social service and drug treatment agencies has received little attention. This is an important avenue of research.

Investigators must evaluate the capacity for programs that have relied on chemotherapeutic interventions alone (MMTP) to deal with both the medical-social problems of HIV/NDU, and drug problems (cocaine/ crack) not currently amenable to chemotherapeutic intervention. We must learn how the switch to cocaine and "crack" as the drugs of choice has affected treatment potential for the NDU.

CONCLUSION

Clearly, community-based social services (linked closely with health services) for the NDU with symptomatic HIV disease present a challenge to policymakers and service providers. While NDUs are dying sicker and quicker from AIDS than people infected by other means, this trend may not continue. Through participation in experimental drug trials, such as those for AZT, and creation of a strong supportive care network, the lives of NDUs with AIDS may be prolonged. The increased prevalence of the disease underscores the need for augmentation of resources and new care and service arrangements. Without systematic planning, thousands of NDUs will remain outside the health and social service systems. With creativity, however, perhaps another 20 percent or more of the currently untreated addicts can be successfully engaged and treated.

The Nation's consciousness and sense of humanity relative to the AIDS epidemic will be the driving force behind our willingness to allocate adequate financial resources and encourage the development of alternative structures and new modes of service delivery. History tells us that change is often precipitated by socioeconomic crises (resulting from war and disease) and people's reactive values and attitudes rather than incremental planning. With AIDS, the pendulum is still swinging. Will people be more compassionate and strongly voice their support for increased resource allocation and service system restructuring? Or will Puritanism and condemnatory social and health policies prevail?

REFERENCES

Axthelm, P. Somebody else's kids. *Newsweek*, April 25, 1988. pp. 64-68.

Balian, P.; Lebouc, V.; Roustang, I.; Bouchard, I.; Polo de Voto, J.; and Espinoza, P. Has the open sale of syringes modified the syringe exchanging habits of I.V.D.A. Poster session presented at the Fourth International Conference on AIDS, Stockholm, Sweden, June 1988.

Barton, E. Vice President for Administration, Samaritan Village, New York, NY. Personal communication, 1988.

Belmont, M.; Mantell, J.; and Spivak, H. *Resource Utilization by AIDS Patients in the Acute Care Hospital.* Final report to the Health Services Improvement Fund, Inc., Empire Blue Cross/Blue Shield, New York, NY, December 1985. 197 pp.

Brager, G., and Hollaway, S. *Changing Human Service Organizations: Politics and Practice.* New York: The Free Press, 1978. 244 pp.

Campbell, G. Director, Division of AIDS Services, Office of Home Care Services, New York City Human Resources Administration. Personal communication, 1987.

Carpi, J. Housing IV drug users who have not kicked the habit. *AIDS Patient Care*, April 1988.

Centers for Disease Control, AIDS Program, Center for Infectious Diseases. *AIDS Weekly Surveillance Report–United States*, November 28, 1988.

Centers for Disease Control. Human immunodeficiency virus infection in the United States: A review of current knowledge. *MMWR* 36 (suppl. no. S-6):1-48, December 18, 1987.

Check, W. Beyond the political modeling of reporting: Nonspecific symptoms in media communication about AIDS. *Rev Infect Dis* 9:987-1000, 1987.

Cohen, J. Director, AWARE Program, University of California at San Francisco. Personal communication, 1987.

Cohen, J.; Hauer, L.; and Wofsey, C. Women and IV drugs: Parenteral and heterosexual transmission of human immunodeficiency virus. *J Drug Issues*, in press.

Daley, S. Runaways of 42nd street: AIDS begins its scourge. *New York Times*, May 30, 1988. p. 25.

Froner, G. AIDS and homelessness. *J Psychoactive Drugs* 20:197-202, April-June 1988.

Goffman, E. *Asylums.* Garden City: Doubleday/Anchor Books, 1967.

Grieco, M.H. Director, Infectious Diseases and Epidemiology, St. Luke's-Roosevelt Hospital Center, New York, NY. Personal communication, 1988.

Gross, J. Needle exchange for addicts wins foothold against AIDS in Tacoma. *New York Times*, January 23, 1989. p. A12.

Guinan, M., and Hardy, A. Epidemiology of AIDS in women in the United States. *JAMA* 257:2039-2042, 1987.

Hegarty, J.D.; Abrams, E.J.; Hutchinson, V.E.; Nicholas, S.W.; Suarez, M.S.; and Heagarty, M.C. The medical care costs of human immunodeficiency virus-infected children in Harlem. *JAMA* 260:1901-1905, 1984.

Hein, K. AIDS in adolescence: a rationale for concern. Paper prepared for the Council on Adolescent Development of the Carnegie Corporation, April 1988. 68 pp.

Kemper, K., and Forsyth, B. Medically unnecessary hospital use in children seropositive for human immunodeficiency virus. *JAMA* 260:1906-1909, October 7, 1988.

Kerr, P. Concerns about AIDS and crime spurring push to expand drug treatment programs. *New York Times*, September 7, 1988. p. A18.

Lambert, B. AIDS danger rises for cocaine users. *New York Times*, November 28, 1988a. p. A2.

Lambert, B. Panel asks for major expansion of drug clinics to combat AIDS. *New York Times*, September 16, 1988b. pp. B1, B7.

Lewis, B.; Sullivan, J.; McCusker, J.; Birch, F.; Koblin, B.; and Hagan, H. Comprehensive surveillance of HIV among IVDUs in Worcester, Massachusetts. Poster presented at the Fourth International Conference on AIDS, Stockholm, Sweden, June 1988.

Maayan, F.; Wormser, G.; Hewlett, D.; Miller, S.; Duncanson, F.; Rodriguez, A.; Perla, E.N.; Koppel, B.; and Rieber, E.E. Acquired immunodeficiency syndrome (AIDS) in an economically disadvantaged population. *Arch Intern Med* 145:1607-1612, 1985.

Marlink, R.; Foss, B.; Swift, R.; Davis, W.; and Essex, M. High rate of HTLV-III/HIV exposure in IVDAs from a small-sized city and the failure of methadone maintenance to prevent further drug use. Paper presented at the Third International Conference on AIDS, Washington, DC, June 1987.

Mondanaro, J. *Chemically Dependent Women--Assessment and Treatment*. Lexington, MA: Lexington Books, 1989. 170 pp.

Mulleady, G.; Roderick, P.; Flanagan, D.; Burnyeat, S.; Wade, B.; Clarke, H.; and McAught, A. HIV and drug abuse: Essential factors in providing a syringe exchange service. Poster session presented at the Fourth International Conference on AIDS, Stockholm, Sweden, June 1988.

New York City Department of Health, AIDS Surveillance Unit. *AIDS Surveillance Update*, January 25, 1989.

New York Times. Editorial: Contain AIDS by treating addicts. January 31, 1988a. p. 26.

New York Times. Editorial: Beyond needles: The AIDS war. February 11, 1988b. p. A34.

Norman, C. Health problems of the homeless. *Science* 242:188-189, October 14, 1988.

Novick, L.F.; Berns, D.; Stricof, R.; and Stevens, R. HIV seroprevalence in newborn infants in New York State. Paper presented at the American Public Health Association Meeting, Boston, MA, November 1988.

Rothenberg, R.; Woelfel, M.; Stoneburner, R.; Milberg, J.; Parker, R.; and Truman, B. Survival with the acquired immunodeficiency syndrome. *New Engl J Med* 317:1297-1302, 1987.

San Francisco Department of Public Health. *AIDS in San Francisco: Status Report for Fiscal Year 1987-88 and Projections of Service Needs and Costs for 1988-93.* San Francisco Department of Public Health, San Francisco, CA, April 22, 1988. 283 pp.

Schmalz, J. Addicts to get needles in plan to curb AIDS. *New York Times*, January 31, 1988. pp. 1, 36.

Shulman, L. Social work practice and the revolutions in health care. Keynote Address, National Association of Perinatal Social Workers, New Orleans, LA, May 24, 1985.

Sorrell, S. Medical Director, Substance Abuse Program, St. Luke's-Roosevelt Hospital Center, New York, NY. Personal communication, 1988.

Stoneburner, R.L.; Des Jarlais, D.C.; Benezra, D.; Gorelkin, L.; Sotheran, J.L.; Friedman, S.R.; Schultz, S.; Marmor, M.; Mildvan, D.; and Maslansky, R. A larger spectrum of severe HIV-1-related disease in intravenous drug users in New York City. *Science* 242:916-919, November 10, 1988.

U.S. Department of Health and Human Services. *Fiscal Year 1985 Study of Runaways and Youth.* Washington, DC, 1986.

Vernick, J. Clinical Director, Baker Places, Inc., San Francisco, CA. Personal communication, April 1987.

Wilensky, H., and Lebeaux, C. *Industrial Society and Social Welfare.* New York: The Free Press, 1965. 397 pp.

AUTHORS

Lawrence C. Shulman, M.S.W., A.C.S.W.
Vice President for Social Work
St. Luke's-Roosevelt Hospital Center
428 West 59th Street
New York, NY 10019
                    and
Adjunct Associate Professor
Columbia University School of Social Work
622 West 113th Street
New York, NY 10025

Joanne E. Mantell, Ph.D., M.S.P.H.
Senior Research Scientist
New York City Department of Health
Director and Principal Investigator, Prevention
    of Perinatal HIV Infection and AIDS Community
    Demonstration Project
AIDS Research Unit, Box A/1
125 Worth Street
New York, NY 10013
                     and
Principal Investigator, AIDS Behavioral Research Program
Gay Men's Health Crisis
Education Department
129 West 20th Street
New York, NY 10011

Charles Eaton, M.S.
Coordinator
Needle Exchange Program
New York City Department of Health
AIDS Research Unit
125 Worth Street
New York, NY 10013

Stephan Sorrell, M.D.
Medical Director, Substance Abuse Program
St. Luke's-Roosevelt Hospital Center
428 West 59th Street
New York, NY 10019

Accessing Intravenous Drug Users via the Health Care System

Patricia E. Evans

INTRODUCTION

The acquired immunodeficiency syndrome (AIDS) epidemic in San Francisco has been an enigma since the first cases were described in 1981. This enigma has continued into 1988 and must be clearly understood to understand the unique differences that exist between San Francisco and other areas of the country. For example, the epidemic in San Francisco is largely a disease affecting gay and bisexual men and has continued as such since the beginning of the epidemic in 1981. Of the 4,371 total AIDS cases reported in San Francisco as of 31 January 1988, 4,212 cases, or 97 percent, are gay/bisexual men, of whom 520, or 11.9 percent, are also intravenous drug users (IVDUs), while 3,681 cases, or 84 percent, are white (San Francisco Department of Public Health 1988a). Nationally, 52,256 cases were reported to the Centers for Disease Control (CDC) as of 1 February 1988, of whom 37,227, or 72 percent, were gay/ bisexual males. Of these, 3,858, or 8 percent, were IVDUs. In contrast to the local statistics, 31,283, or only 61 percent nationally, were white (Centers for Disease Control 1988).

In San Francisco, the number of heterosexual IVDUs is 62, or 1.4 percent of the total caseload. In contrast, the number of heterosexual IVDUs nationally is 8,877, or 17 percent.

MINORITIES AND AIDS

A closer review of minorities with AIDS in the United States illustrates the stark realities of the disproportionate number of cases among blacks and Hispanics, as depicted in tables 1 through 6.

TABLE 1. *AIDS in blacks and Hispanics (n=44,767)*

Blacks and Hispanics	Percent of AIDS Cases
Total	39
Women	70
Heterosexuals	71
Children	77

NOTE: Cases reported to CDC by 2 November 1987.

Tables 2 and 3 provide a closer review of AIDS cases by transmission category for ethnic groups.

TABLE 2. *AIDS cases by transmission category and ethnic group (percent)*

	White (n=22,299)	Black (n=7,729)	Hispanic (n=4,373)
Gay/Bisexual– Non-IVDU	82.8	47.5	54.5
IVDU or Sex Partner of IVDU	12.3	40.1	40.4
Other	4.9	12.4	5.1

A look at the IV-drug-using population in the United States and San Francisco is depicted in table 5.

As can be seen, the percentage of AIDS cases associated with IV drug use in San Francisco is lower in all categories with the exception of gay/bisexual males, who have used IV drugs (8 percent vs. 12 percent) (Centers for Disease Control 1988; San Francisco Department of Public Health 1988a).

TABLE 3. *AIDS cases by transmission category comparing ethnic groups (percent)*

	White (n=739)	Black (n=1,314)	Hispanic (n=446)
IVDU or Sex Partners of IVDUs	47.8	69.9	82.5
Sex Partner of Bisexual Men	6.9	2.8	2.7
Other Women with AIDS	45.3	27.3	14.8

TABLE 4. *AIDS cases in children by transmission category comparing ethnic groups (percent)*

	White (n=117)	Black (n=283)	Hispanic (n=107)
Mother or Mother's Sex Partner was IVDU	39.8	60.8	5.7
Other Children with AIDS	60.2	39.2	24.3

SOURCE: Centers for Disease Control 1987.

CHARACTERISTICS OF IVDUs IN SAN FRANCISCO

There are an estimated 10,000 to 12,000 IVDUs in San Francisco (Newmeyer 1987). The racial composition of IVDUs in drug abuse treatment in 1985 to 1986 and 1986 to 1987 is presented in table 6.

In the period 1986 to 1987, 38 percent of the IVDUs in San Francisco were female and 62 percent were male. Sixty-eight percent, or 5,651 IVDUs were admitted for heroin use, 6 percent, or 460 for

TABLE 5. *Comparison of AIDS case distribution for selected risk groups, United States vs. San Francisco (percent)*

Risk Group	United States (n=51,467)	San Francisco (n=4,371)
Heterosexual IVDUs as Percent of All Adult AIDS Cases	17	8.5
Gay/Bisexual Male IVDUs as Percent of All Adult AIDS Cases	8	12
Female Sex Partners of IVDUs as Percent of All Female Hetero-sexual Cases	80	46
Children Born to IVDUs or Their Sex Partners as Percent of All Perinatal AIDS Cases	75	54

TABLE 6. *Racial composition of IVDUs in treatment in San Francisco, 1985 to 1986 and 1986 to 1987 (percent)*

Race	1985-86 (n=5,800)	1986-87 (n=8,232)
White	58	52
Black	23	28
Latino	15	14
Asian	3	5
Native American	1	1

SOURCE: San Francisco Department of Public Health 1988b.

amphetamine use, and 13 percent, or 1,045 for cocaine use (San Francisco Department of Public Health 1987).

There are indications that the IV-drug-using populations in San Francisco are at increasing risk of developing AIDS, especially when seropositivity data are analyzed. These data indicate that, over time, there has been a slow but steady increase in human immuno-deficiency virus (HIV) seropositivity, especially among the ethnic minority IV-drug-using populations. Chaisson and colleagues have followed IVDUs in treatment since 1984, and their data, presented in table 7, demonstrate these increases (Chaisson et al. 1988).

TABLE 7. *HIV seropositivity rates in heterosexual IVDUs*

	Treatment Programs			Hospitalized Users		
Year	HIV Sero-positive	IVDUs	Percent	HIV Sero-positive	IVDUs	Percent
1983-84	3	77	4	3	21	14
1985	22	234	12		N/A	
1986-87	96	764	13	8	44	18

Watters, of the Urban Health Project, has provided information regarding the IVDUs not in treatment. His figures for 1986 range from 7 percent for IVDUs participating in a 21-day detoxification program to 16 percent for IVDUs not in treatment (Watters 1987). Chaisson's data, broken down by ethnic group, are presented in table 8.

HEALTH CARE SYSTEMS

There has been a greater increase for the black IV-drug-using community than for other groups. Consequently, the door is open for a significant increase in HIV infection and AIDS among heterosexual IVDUs to emerge in San Francisco unless effective strategies to prevent further spread among IVDUs are in place and working effectively.

TABLE 8. *HIV seropositivity rates by ethnic group for heterosexual IVDUs in treatment (percent)*

Ethnic Group	1985	1986–87
White	143 (6%)	328 (7%)
Black	60 (15%)	188 (26%)
Hispanic	78 (14%)	94 (10%)

First, we must ask ourselves if we intend to solve this epidemic using known public health methods, which are global in nature, or if we will use the political, or band-aid, approach.

Since I have been asked to focus on the health care delivery system and how to reach the IV-drug-using population, let me provide some background information. In general, the health care system can be described as a huge and complex system within systems, which can be divided into the public and the private sectors.

The private sector consists of health care providers in private practice, members of health maintenance organizations (HMOs), preferred provider organizations (PPOs), Independent Practice Associations (IPAs), and other alphabetical abbreviations, so commonplace today. Various hospital systems, for profit or not for profit, are also included in the private sector share of the health care system. Although there are IVDUs who use the private system, the vast majority of highest risk IVDUs do not generally receive services from this part of the health care system.

The public sector includes public hospitals, public clinics, and other public health care facilities and services, such as laboratories, immunizations, or environmental health.

For our purposes, health care services incorporate all health services including public health. "Public health services exist primarily to prevent disease, promote health, and to measure and evaluate the health status of populations" (Last 1980, p. 3). By taking a global approach to the AIDS epidemic, good public health measures can certainly assist in the war against this deadly disease.

Prevention Via the Public Health System

Preventive services, which form a large part of public health, can be broken down as follows:

- Community services—those aimed at the community (e.g., clean water);

- Personal services—those aimed at the individual (e.g., health education and risk reduction for smoking cessation); and

- Combined community and personal services—those aimed at both the community and the individual (e.g., screening or immunizations) (Jonas 1980).

Prevention can be further categorized as primary, secondary, or tertiary (Last 1980). Primary prevention deals with preventing the occurrence of disease or injury (e.g., by immunization). Since there is no vaccine currently available for AIDS, primary prevention does not seem likely in the very near future.

Secondary prevention deals with early detection and intervention (e.g., HIV antibody screening, health education, and counseling of seropositive individuals.)

Tertiary prevention deals with minimizing the effects of disease and disability by surveillance and maintenance aimed at preventing complications and deterioration (e.g., use of AZT in asymptomatic HIV-positive individuals).

A major question to ask is: How can the IVDU be reached through the current health care system from a public health, preventive perspective?

Figure 1 is a very complicated diagram of perinatal services in San Francisco. Although complex, it can be viewed as an excellent example of reaching IVDUs. As can be noted, many of the programs listed are actually prevention programs. Many public health departments have moved away from the prevention-only model to providing primary care in public health clinics. The hospital system is a prime example of a model that combines primary, secondary, and tertiary care required for medically indigent adults as well as those individuals requiring care through the public health system. Many contacts with IVDUs may be secondary or peripheral to the IVDU, because the primary contact is with the sexual partner of the IVDU or other family members. These opportunities must be seized and utilized to the greatest advantage. Thus, unique opportunities for providing education and prevention do exist.

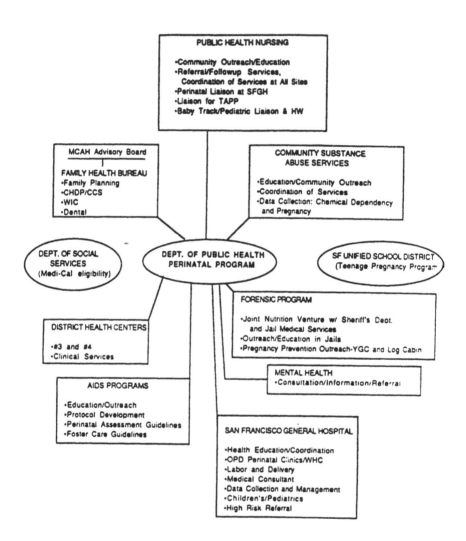

FIGURE 1. *Perinatal program links*

SOURCE: San Francisco Department of Health 1987.

Utilizing Prevention/Education Opportunities

Public health nursing is often called upon to assist in a clearer understanding of family dynamics related to certain circumstances (e.g., child abuse, family dysfunction, or inappropriate use of the health care system.) During these family or home visits, the public health nurse is instrumental in obtaining significant information that may assist providers in understanding the family situation and the reason behind certain types of behavior. These encounters can assist in identifying high-risk individuals and can also provide opportunities for education and referral of high-risk persons.

District health centers provide primary care as well as preventive care to families and individuals seeking services from the public health care system. Thus, there is opportunity for direct contact with the IVDU or with family members within these centers.

Preventive programs such as WIC (Women, Infant, and Children Feeding Program), CHDP (Child Health and Disability Prevention Program), and immunizations allow for repeated contacts with family members, during which brief educational messages can be imparted.

The Forensic Program allows direct access to jail inmates, male and female, and again provides opportunities for individual and group educational interventions with IVDUs and their sex partners.

The hospital system provides for a variety of needs for the clients seeking care through this system. Although usually overburdened and overworked, it can provide a setting to reach IVDUs at many levels (San Francisco Department of Public Health 1987).

STRATEGIES FOR DEVELOPING HEALTH CARE SYSTEMS

Although these are only a few examples of how to reach the at-risk populations, this model can be developed for most public health programs. There are a number of steps that must be taken to make this type of system effective, however, if behavior change of the at-risk population is the ultimate goal.

Full education of health care providers working in the system is needed to enlighten providers regarding AIDS, its prevention, transmission, etc. Too often, it is assumed that knowledge about a new development or disease will be acquired automatically by those caring for the ill. This assumption is a fallacy; education must be afforded health care providers to assist them in gaining the knowledge to become more comfortable with a disease process.

Since AIDS touches upon subjects often taboo in society (sexuality and IV drug use), providers' prejudices regarding these subjects must be dealt with in an open and forthright manner.

Because IVDUs and minorities are so closely linked with AIDS, providers' prejudices relating to social deviance, sexism, and racism must be dealt with openly, and opportunities for understanding one's feeling in relationship to this disease must be given.

There must be better education of students of health care and health care professionals, so that they clearly understand drug abuse, treatment modalities, and the whys and wherefores of intervention programs.

Providers must become comfortable with taking sexual and drug histories in a nonjudgmental fashion with all clients entering and participating in the health care system, not just those considered to be at risk. Assumptions about one's probability of being infected should not enter into history taking. But a good history will assist in identifying additional patients who could be at risk.

There must be a clear understanding of the entire health care system and where, throughout the system, efforts can be made effectively to change a client's behavior and allow positive reinforcement of behavior change.

Informal or formal links must be developed between programs to allow for ease of referral.

Last, additional monies must be added to an already overburdened and overwhelmed system. AIDS has pushed the system to the limits and will continue to do so. Therefore, additional funding must be added to the system to prevent total collapse. Other prevention programs cannot be allowed to fall by the wayside at the expense of those who are already infected, ill, and dying.

REFERENCES

Centers for Disease Control. Minority Slides (1-238). Center for Infectious Diseases, Centers for Disease Control, November 2, 1987.

Centers for Disease Control. *AIDS Surveillance Report - United States AIDS Program.* Center for Infectious Diseases, Centers for Disease Control, February 1988.

Chaisson, R.; Bacchetti, P.; Osmond, D.; Brodi, B.; Sande, M.; and Moss, A. HIV infection in intravenous drug users in San Francisco. Presented by Andrew Moss, M.D., at the Center for AIDS Prevention Studies Community Forum on AIDS Education Interventions for IVDUs, February 1988.

Jonas, J. Provision of public health services. In: Last, J.M., ed. *Public Health and Preventive Medicine.* New York: Appleton, Century-Crofts, 1980. pp. 1614-1633.

Last, J.M. Scope and methods of prevention. In: Last, J.M., ed. *Public Health and Preventive Medicine.* New York: Appleton, Century-Crofts, 1980. pp. 3-8.

Newmeyer, J. Personal communication, 1987.

San Francisco Department of Public Health. *Perinatal Plan, FY 1987-88.* Report to Health Commission, City and County of San Francisco, January 1987.

San Francisco Department of Public Health. *Acquired Immunodeficiency Syndrome (AIDS) Monthly Surveillance Report: Summary of Cases Meeting the CDC Surveillance Definition in San Francisco Cases Reported through 1/31/88.* 1988a.

San Francisco Department of Public Health, Division of Mental Health, Substance Abuse and Forensic Services. *Community Substance Abuse Services Updated Plan for Fiscal Year 1988-89.* Draft, 1988b.

Watters, J.K. Preventing human immunodeficiency virus contagion among intravenous drug users: The impact of street-based education on risk behavior. Presented at the Third International Conference on AIDS, Washington, DC, June 1-5, 1987.

AUTHOR

Patricia E. Evans, M.D., M.P.H.
Associate Medical Director
AIDS Office, San Francisco
1111 Market Street, 3rd Floor
San Francisco, CA 94103

Community Prevention Efforts to Reduce the Spread of AIDS Associated With Intravenous Drug Abuse

Robert J. Battjes, Carl G. Leukefeld, and Zili Amsel

Developing an effective vaccine to prevent the spread of the acquired immunodeficiency syndrome (AIDS) is expected to take a long time, and, until a vaccine is developed, the only means to prevent the spread of AIDS is through behavior change. Therefore, persons at risk for human immunodeficiency virus (HIV) infection must be informed of their risk for AIDS and helped to modify behaviors that place them at risk.

This monograph has focused on the prevention of HIV transmission among intravenous (IV) drug abusers, from drug abusers to their sexual partners, and perinatally to their children. IV drug abuse has played a major role in the spread of the AIDS epidemic. IV drug abusers constitute 30 percent of recently reported adult AIDS cases in the United States (Centers for Disease Control 1988). Also, the heterosexual and perinatal spread of AIDS is largely associated with IV drug abuse (Chamberland et al. 1987; Oxtoby, personal communication, 1987), and IV drug abusers have been identified as major vectors for the spread of AIDS to the general population (U.S. Public Health Service 1986).

The potential for rapid spread of HIV among IV drug abusers exists because such drug abusers commonly share drug injection equipm This rapid spread has been demonstrated in New York City. While the first cases of HIV infection among IV drug abusers appeared there in 1978, 25 percent of a sample of such abusers were infected by 1979, and infection rates approximated 60 percent by late 1986 (Des Jarlais, personal communication, 1987). While high levels of H infection are found among IV drug abusers in New York City and several other major metropolitan areas, infection rates are still low ir

288

many parts of the United States (Hahn et al. 1988). It is crucial that effective AIDS prevention programs be initiated throughout the country to prevent further spread of HIV in high-prevalence areas and to prevent initial spread in low-prevalence areas. IV drug abusers and their sexual partners must be helped to change those behaviors that place them, others, and their unborn children at risk.

Behavior change is often difficult, especially when targeted behaviors are valued and/or reinforced. Yet, many Americans are changing their behaviors to improve their own health—fewer people are smoking; more people are exercising; and many people have reduced fat consumption. These behavior changes within the general U.S. population have been achieved slowly and incrementally over the past few decades, and many Americans continue to smoke, lead sedentary lives, and consume excess fats.

Drug-abusing behaviors—most specifically, needle use—are among those behaviors that have proven difficult to modify. Drug dependence is a chronic medical disorder, not a temporary condition. Overcoming dependence requires extensive lifestyle change, and long-term abstinence is difficult to achieve without help. Even with intensive drug abuse treatment, most IV drug abusers require repeated and prolonged treatment to overcome drug dependence. Short of abstinence from drugs, behavior change to reduce risk of HIV transmission is also difficult to achieve. However, IV drug abusers are generally concerned about their risk for AIDS, and many are taking steps to reduce their risks (Des Jarlais et al. 1988; Newmeyer 1988). Yet, it appears that risk-reduction efforts by drug abusers are often incomplete and inconsistently applied, and many IV drug abusers continue to regularly engage in high-risk behaviors. Sexual behaviors are also difficult to modify and may be even more resistant to change than drug-using behaviors (Newmeyer 1988).

Thus, using behavior change approaches to prevent AIDS associated with IV drug abuse presents a challenge. Providing information alone is not sufficient. It is apparent that IV drug abusers and their sexual partners will need considerable help to consistently and effectively reduce their risks for contracting and transmitting HIV. Considering the urgency of this need, it is essential that AIDS prevention initiatives be designed for maximum effectiveness.

Experiences with other behaviors, such as dietary modification, smoking cessation, and performance of a regular exercise regimen, have shown that both the initiation and the maintenance of behavioral change can be successfully achieved within the context of the target group's environment or community (Fortmann et al. 1986; Pushka et al. 1983). Community prevention approaches are designed for specific target groups, are delivered by individuals and organizations that have credibility and are trusted within the target groups, and incorporate social support within the community to reinforce behavioral change (Nelkin 1987). Thus, rather than relying on a single intervention strategy, community prevention approaches use multiple sources to encourage, support, and reinforce change. Based on the success of community prevention in changing selected health behaviors, this approach provides possible models for designing programs to prevent the spread of AIDS.

Like the general population, IV drug abusers and their sexual partners are members of various well-defined communities. By consolidating knowledge about these communities, their structure, how IV drug abusers and their sexual partners interact with their communities, and how these communities affect behavior, strategies can be developed to reach IV drug abusers and their sexual partners and to help these target groups reduce their risks for contracting and transmitting HIV.

The technical review that served as the basis of this monograph was designed to explore "communities" and their potential as vehicles for the implementation of AIDS prevention strategies aimed at IV drug abusers, their sexual partners, and their children. In the prior chapters, the authors have discussed AIDS prevention issues relevant to various target communities. Some of the communities are distinguished by the demographic characteristics of their memberships. Chapters address specific racial/ethnic groups, women, white males, gay IV drug abusers, nonopiate IV drug abusers, and prostitutes who are IV drug abusers. The monograph also includes communities that are defined by institutional setting. Chapters address schools, drug abuse treatment programs, the criminal justice system, shelters for the homeless, the social service system, and the health care system.

FRAMEWORKS FOR COMMUNITY PREVENTION

Two of the authors, Maccoby and Gilchrist, present frameworks that are useful guides for community AIDS prevention, regardless of the "community" that is being considered. These frameworks will be reviewed briefly before considering the recommendations for community prevention and research that emanated from the technical review.

Maccoby has summarized the experiences of one research team that implemented a series of coordinated community health promotion programs combining the use of media and face-to-face interventions. Several points made by Maccoby in his chapter warrant emphasis here.

First, their research and interventions moved beyond many prevention approaches that focus simply on providing information, modifying attitudes, and motivating behavior change to include teaching target audiences specific behavioral skills in self-regulation (i.e., control over ones own behavior).

Second, they used a sequential strategy that proceeded through specific stages, including the presentation of information, stimulating the development of personal analyses of risk behaviors, and demonstrating desired skills.

Third, knowledge, beliefs, attitudes, risk-related behaviors, and media exposure of their target audience were continuously monitored and their intervention(s) were modified, based on this feedback information.

Fourth, program design proceeded through specific steps and was guided by a formative evaluation that began with a needs analysis of the target audience and proceeded to segment the audience into subsections for program development.

Fifth, local communities were involved in program design from the outset to assure their ownership and control of the program, to take advantage of interpersonal leadership of key individuals, and, thereby, to enhance the likelihood of initial success and program durability.

Another broad framework that is useful in developing community AIDS prevention initiatives was presented by Gilchrist, drawing on the work of R.S. Gordon (1983). This typology for adolescent prevention programming, which is applicable to prevention efforts with other "communities" as well, identifies three levels of program intensity, based on the target groups' risk potential. The first level of programming, "universal," is aimed at the general public. Universal programming, the least intensive level, provides information and opportunity to practice those skills that are needed to maintain safe behavior. The second level of programming, "selective," focuses on geographic areas where the AIDS risk is above average, i.e., areas where drug use, delinquency, and sexually transmitted disease rates are high. Selective programming is more intensive, including additional program elements such as stress management, building self-esteem, and developing communications skills. The third level of programming, "indicated," concentrates on individuals who are already engaging in behavior associated with HIV transmission. Indicated programming must be highly personalized and provide support over an extended time period. Thus, in planning community AIDS prevention programs, it is important to first analyze the degree of risk potential of the community and various segments of the community.

RECOMMENDATIONS

The following recommendations are presented with the general goal of furthering and expanding the current state-of-the-art of community interventions focused on preventing the spread of HIV among IV drug abusers, their sexual partners, and their children. In keeping with the comprehensive purpose of the technical review, to describe innovative community prevention efforts for IV drug abusers, and to specify research initiatives, the recommendations are grouped under two areas: community intervention recommendations and research recommendations. It should be noted that these recommendations do not represent the consensus of those participants who attended the technical review, but they do present general agreement.

Community Intervention Recommendations

- Guiding principles recommended for community intervention programs are as follows: (1) interventions should incorporate multiple and repeated components to increase the likelihood of reaching and having a lasting effect on the target group; (2) interventions cannot be viewed in isolation, but must draw upon other community resources; (3) case management staff are needed to aggressively seek out the target groups (IV drug abusers, their spouses, and other sexual partners) and to link them with relevant community resources; (4) interventions must be intended to reach people where they are—to build on their own motivation, rather than demanding that they behave as society believes they should; and (5) activities related to AIDS transmission cannot be considered in isolation, but must be considered in the context of major social problems, including homelessness, poverty, joblessness, and racism.

- From the public health point of view, and to contain the spread of HIV, it is essential that the goal of drug abuse abstinence and the goal of HIV prevention be recognized as separate issues. Abstinence is the most effective means of HIV prevention, and it is desirable to help IV drug abusers stop using drugs. However, it must be recognized that many IV drug abusers will be unwilling or unable to stop. Thus, interventions with IV drug abusers who are not in treatment should have a dual focus—encouraging risk-reduction efforts and entry into treatment.

- Drug abuse treatment is an important element in community AIDS prevention. A major limitation has been the lack of sufficient treatment availability. In major metropolitan areas where drug abuse is endemic, drug abuse treatment programs are filled to capacity, and addicts seeking treatment are placed on waiting lists or simply turned away. If the potential of drug abuse treatment as an AIDS prevention strategy is to be realized, treatment capacity must be expanded, and additional treatment personnel must be trained to provide these services.

- If the contribution of drug abuse treatment to AIDS prevention is to be maximized, treatment must not only be expanded, but must also be made more flexible and accessible. Same-day intake services should be available to those seeking help, and treatment should be available 24 hours per day. In addition, treatment programs need to reach out into the community. Services must be culturally specific and linguistically appropriate for various target communities.

- Outreach efforts should encourage and facilitate entry into drug abuse treatment for those who are willing, and should encourage other risk-reduction behaviors for those who are not. The expansion of treatment must be accompanied by an expansion of outreach efforts into all areas where IV drug abuse is endemic. Outreach services, using indigenous workers who have credibility and can penetrate drug-abusing subcultures, are an important part of community prevention efforts with drug abusers not in treatment. However, outreach efforts should not rely entirely on indigenous workers—workers with a range of expertise and background experiences are needed. In addition to street outreach, outreach should also occur using other approaches, such as the use of mobile vans in areas where drug abuse is endemic and through various community agencies such as public housing programs, the criminal justice system, hospital emergency rooms, public health centers, sexually transmitted disease clinics, homeless

293

shelters, and single-room-occupancy hotels. Staffs of such agencies should be trained regarding both IV drug abuse and AIDS, and AIDS education should be available to IV drug abusers within these facilities.

- Given the large numbers of IV drug abusers who are involved with the criminal justice system, lockups, jails, prisons, and probation and parole offices can provide important access points for AIDS education to encourage behavior change and to facilitate referral to drug abuse treatment. Linkages between the criminal justice system and drug abuse treatment should facilitate initiation of treatment prior to institutional discharge and provide for the ongoing involvement of probation and parole officials in support of the treatment process.

- Specific outreach programs are needed for the various special target communities addressed earlier in this monograph, such as blacks, Hispanics, women, gays, and the homeless. And there is a need to target subsegments of these communities, such as pregnant women. Homeless drug abusers provide an example of a target community that will need an array of supportive social services if AIDS prevention services are to be effective. AIDS risk behaviors and housing problems are intertwined--the needs of homeless IV drug abusers for adequate housing must be addressed if AIDS risk reduction is to be achieved and maintained. Similarly, for many target groups, health care services play an important role in community AIDS prevention by providing a locus for interventions and supporting behavior change efforts. Community-based, multi-service centers are necessary to provide adequate health care to supplement drug abuse treatment programs in order to meet the health care needs of IV drug abusers.

- Prevention efforts cannot focus on IV drug abusers only, but must also reach their sexual partners. As with IV drug abusers themselves, prevention efforts aimed at sexual partners must utilize indigenous workers and community agencies that currently are in contact with this group. It is especially important that supportive services for women offer alternatives to unprotected, unsafe sex. Prevention efforts should also target families of IV drug abusers, so that family members encourage and support behavior change.

- Community AIDS prevention efforts must focus not simply on those who are not yet infected, but also on those who are already infected, in order to reduce their likelihood of transmitting HIV to others. Messages for those infected need to communicate—"Living with HIV infection, not dying from AIDS."

- Finally, major barriers to community interventions were identified. These included the lack of adequate funding for drug abuse treatment and AIDS outreach, community opposition to the expansion of drug abuse services, fragmentation of services, fees for treatment that deter treatment entry, lack of appropriately trained personnel to provide treatment and outreach, lack of leadership at all levels, and existence of paraphernalia laws that prevent exploration of needle distribution approaches.

Research Recommendations

Community research in the drug abuse field is in its infancy. Success with community interventions focused on selected health behaviors are encouraging, yet the promise of community approaches in preventing the spread of HIV infection among IV drug abusers, their sexual partners, and children is as yet untested. Thus, a rigorous program of research is needed to develop effective interventions. The review group made a number of recommendations relevant to community interventions. These recommendations touched on the need for data to guide interventions as well as outcome research to determine program efficacy.

- Research is needed on the incidence and prevalence of HIV infection among IV drug abusers and their sexual partners to better define the target populations. Changes in prevalence over time must also be determined to understand the spread of the epidemic.

- Research should focus on risk behaviors. What are these behaviors? What is the prevalence and incidence of these behaviors? What is their meaning? What factors support the maintenance of risk behaviors? How are behaviors changing in response to the AIDS epidemic?

- Research should focus on community or population traits that support or impede behavior change. What are community attitudes, norms, values, or other cultural characteristics that affect risk behaviors and efforts to change behaviors? What community support systems and communication patterns affect efforts to change risk behaviors?

- Research should focus on community information channels. What networks, resources, and services have credibility?

- At the community level, evaluative research needs to determine baseline measures of risk behaviors, HIV infection, and AIDS and determine the changes in these measures over time. Community interventions need to be theory-based and adapted to the needs of the specific community through developmental research. Project implementation should be designed to permit evaluation of program models, including process evaluation (e.g., availability, accept-ability, satisfaction) and outcome evaluation (e.g., changes in knowledge and attitudes, risk behaviors, and incidence of HIV infection).

A number of methodological issues affect the ability to evaluate community interventions. These issues are not unique to AIDS prevention initiatives, but are common to all community prevention research efforts. A major drawback to efforts to "prove" that community prevention approaches are effective may be a lack of appropriate research methods to demonstrate a program effect. Specific methodological issues identified include the following:

- One issue is the difficulty in measuring effect. HIV infection, the ultimate measure of program effect, may not be a sensitive indicator, especially in areas where infection rates are initially very low. Measurement of highly personal and illegal risk behaviors such as sexual intercourse and IV drug abuse must generally rely on subject self-report, which raises issues of the validity of the outcome data.

- Other issues relate to the use of appropriate control or comparison groups in community research. Randomization of subjects to treatment conditions is seldom possible. Random assignment of communities to treatment conditions does not assure comparability across conditions except in very large studies where a large number of communities are involved. Comparison commu-nities may be used, but comparability between experimental and comparison communities cannot be assured. Change within a community over time might be assessed, but such a historical control is particularly questionable in the rapidly changing AIDS field.

■ Another issue is the independence of the evaluation. Is the evaluation internal (i.e., conducted by the organization implementing the intervention) or is it external (i.e., conducted by an independent group)? If the evaluation is internal, is there an independent advisory group or some other mechanism to assure the objectivity of the evaluation?

■ A final issue concerns generalizability of research findings. Interventions may not generalize between high- and low-risk communities or across subgroups of a community. Thus, multisite studies and studies focusing on multiple subgroups may be necessary.

A common problem facing both program implementation and research is the definition of the community. To develop effective interventions and to demonstrate their effectiveness require clarity regarding the target community. Too often, community interventions have a vague sense of community—often defined as residents of a certain geographical area. In this review of community AIDS prevention, a number of distinct communities have been identified and considered. While a community intervention may cover multiple communities, the intervention strategies employed must be tailored to the unique needs and resources of the component communities, and research must address program effect on each of these communities.

REFERENCES

Battjes, R.J., and Pickens, R.W., eds. *Needle Sharing Among Intravenous Drug Abusers: National and International Perspectives.* National Institute on Drug Abuse Research Monograph 80. DHHS Pub. No. (ADM)88-1567. Washington, DC: Supt. of Docs., U.S. Govt. Print. Off., 1988. 189 pp.

Centers for Disease Control. *AIDS Weekly Surveillance Report - United States.* Atlanta, GA, October 3, 1988.

Chamberland, M.; White, C.; Lifson, A.; and Dondero, T.J. AIDS in heterosexual contacts: A small but interesting group of cases. Paper presented at Third International Conference on AIDS, Washington, DC, 1987.

Des Jarlais, D.C. New York State Division of Substance Abuse Services, personal communication, 1987.

Des Jarlais, D.C.; Friedman, S.R.; Sotheran, J.L.; and Stoneburner, R. The sharing of drug injection equipment and the AIDS epidemic in New York City: The first decade. In: Battjes, R.J., and Pickens, R.W., eds. *Needle Sharing Among Intravenous Drug Abusers: National and International Perspectives*. National Institute on Drug Abuse Research Monograph 80. DHHS Pub. No. (ADM)88-1567. Washington, DC: Supt. of Docs., U.S. Govt. Print. Off., 1988. pp. 160-175.

Fortmann, S.P.; Haskell, W.L.; Williams, P.T.; Varady, A.N.; Hulley, A.B.; and Farquhar, J.W. Community surveillance of cardiovascular disease in the Stanford Five-City Project: Methods and initial experience. *Am J Epidemiol* 123(4):656-669, 1986.

Gordon, R.S., Jr. An operational classification of disease prevention. *Public Health Rep* 98:107-109, 1983.

Hahn, R.A.; Onorato, I.M.; Jones, T.S.; and Dougherty, J. Infection with human immunodeficiency virus (HIV) among intravenous drug users. Paper presented at Fourth International Conference on AIDS, Stockholm, Sweden, June 1988.

Nelkin, D. AIDS and the social sciences: Review of useful knowledge and research needs. *Rev Infec Dis* 9(5):980-986, 1987.

Newmeyer, J.A. Why bleach? Development of a strategy to combat HIV contagion among San Francisco intravenous drug users. In: Battjes, R.J., and Pickens, R.W., eds. *Needle Sharing Among Intravenous Drug Abusers: National and International Perspectives*. National Institute on Drug Abuse Research Monograph 80. DHHS Pub. No. (ADM)88-1567. Washington, DC: Supt. of Docs., U.S. Govt. Print. Off., 1988. pp. 151-159, 1988.

Oxtoby, M. Centers for Disease Control, personal communication, 1987.

Pushka, P.; Salonen, J.A.; Nissinen, A.; Tuomilehto, J.; Vartiainen, E.; Korhene, H.; Tanskanen, A.; Rönnqvist, P.; Koskela, K.; and Huttunen, J. Change in risk factors for coronary heart disease during 10 years of a community intervention programme. (North Karelia Project) *Br Med J* 287:1840-1844, 1983.

U.S. Public Health Service. Coolfont report: A PHS plan for prevention and control of AIDS and the AIDS virus. *Public Health Rep* 101:341-348, 1986.

AUTHORS

Robert J. Battjes, D.S.W.
Associate Director for Planning

Carl G. Leukefeld, D.S.W.
Deputy Director

Zili Amsel, Sc.D.
Research Epidemiologist
Division of Clinical Research
National Institute on Drug Abuse
Parklawn Building, Rooms 10A38 and 10A16
5600 Fishers Lane
Rockville, MD 20857